Joan Webster
Nutrition.

DEPARTMENT OF HEALTH AND SOCIAL SECURITY

Reports on Public Health and Medical Subjects

No. 120

Recommended Intakes
of Nutrients
for the United Kingdom

(Report of the Panel on Recommended Allowances of Nutrients)

LONDON
HER MAJESTY'S STATIONERY OFFICE
1969: Reprinted 1973

ISBN 0 11 320177 X

ii

CONTENTS

PREFACE

It is over 18 years since the British Medical Association's Committee on Nutrition of 1950 produced their Recommended Allowances. Since then many other countries have brought out analogous tables but this country has remained silent. The delay has not been for want of scientists willing to play their part. Rather, it has reflected the difficulty of their problem as expressed by the Expert Panel on Requirements of Protein, Calcium and other Nutrients of the Committee on Medical and Nutritional Aspects of Food Policy*, which, in 1960, reported that "there is a good deal of ground for suggesting that the recommendations of the BMA need to be revised but we find no basis for immediate revision of them".

The new Panel on Recommended Allowances of Nutrients has now faced this task and this report is the outcome. The authors have been careful to point out that "Recommendations for intakes of nutrients can only be made by the exercise of judgment on limited data; in consequence they can only be provisional and subject to future revision in the light of new knowledge or change of circumstances", and in paragraph 6 they say of the recommendations that "By themselves they cannot be used for the assessment of nutritional status . . .".

Despite such warnings tables of recommended intakes or allowances have often been misinterpreted or misused in the past. In this report recommended intakes are clearly defined as "sufficient or more than sufficient for the nutritional needs of practically all healthy persons in a population". The recommendations for nutrients other than energy must not be equated with requirements; an intake below the recommended levels does not establish the existence of any departure whatever from good health, although its identification may serve a useful purpose by indicating "potential nutritional problems which merit further investigation".

The Committee has been concerned for many years with such nutritional problems. But nutrition in Britain is generally good, and research needed to investigate intakes which do not meet recommended levels is, for technical and practical reasons, difficult and often inconclusive because of the lack of clear objective signs and of the difficulty in securing public participation over long periods. Nevertheless, whatever we can do to ascertain whether deficiencies exist and if so which groups of the population are vulnerable should be done. There may still be ground to be gained by changes in food policy and there is still much uncertainty about the validity of recommended levels of intake.

---

* Now the Committee on Medical Aspects of Food Policy.

The members of this panel have made the most accurate assessment that they can in the light of the available evidence after devoting great trouble and thought to it. Their views on a most complex subject deserve close attention, not least because of the candour with which they have set down the limitations of their authority. As Chairman of the main Committee I record its thanks to the members of the panel, and on behalf of the Health Departments their indebtedness to the members of the Committee for this further contribution to knowledge in a most difficult field.

G. E. GODBER
Chief Medical Officer

MEMBERSHIP OF THE PANEL

Chairman

Dr. R. Passmore — Physiology Department, University of Edinburgh

Members

Dr. W. T. C. Berry — Department of Health and Social Security, London

Dr. A. N. Exton-Smith — Geriatric Department, University College Hospital, London

Miss Dorothy F. Hollingsworth — Ministry of Agriculture, Fisheries and Food, London

Dr. E. Kodicek — Dunn Nutritional Laboratory, Cambridge

Dr. T. E. Oppé — Paediatric Unit, St. Mary's Hospital Medical School, London

Dr. D. S. Parsons — Department of Biochemistry, University of Oxford

Professor B. S. Platt — London School of Hygiene and Tropical Medicine, London

Dr. Elsie M. Widdowson — Dunn Nutritional Laboratory, Cambridge

Professor F. G. Young — Department of Biochemistry, University of Cambridge

Professor J. Yudkin — Queen Elizabeth College, London

Secretariat

Dr. J. P. Greaves (Scientific) — Ministry of Agriculture, Fisheries and Food, London

Dr. Joan M. L. Stephen (Scientific) — Department of Health and Social Security, London

Dr. Joan M. Firth (Administrative) — Department of Health and Social Security, London

The views expressed in this Report are those of the Panel. The valuable help and expert advice received from the following are gratefully acknowledged:
Dr. A. E. Bender, Dr. K. J. Carpenter, Dr. Betty L. Coles, Dr. J. Crooks, Dr. Ethel M. Cruickshank, Professor C. E. Dent, Dr. J. V. G. A. Durnin, Dr. O. G. Edholm, Dr. P. C. Elwood, Professor L. P. R. Fourman, Dr. J. S. Garrow, Dr. E. M. Lawson, Dr. J. Marks, Mr. J. B. Mason, Professor E. M. McGirr, Mr. D. S. Miller, Dr. T. Moore, Dr. D. B. Morgan, Dr. D. Naismith, Mr. P. R. Payne, Dr. H. M. Sinclair, Dr. D. A. T. Southgate, Dr. A. M. Thomson, Dr. W. R. Trotter, Dr. G. R. Wadsworth, Dr. R. G. Whitehead, Professor G. M. Wilson.

RECOMMENDED INTAKES OF NUTRIENTS FOR THE UNITED KINGDOM

INTRODUCTION

1. People vary in their needs for energy and nutrients even after factors such as body size, sex and occupation have been taken into account. The quantity of any nutrient required may also depend on the quality of the diet because the efficiency with which nutrients are absorbed and utilized by the body is influenced by the composition and nature of the diet as a whole.

2. Tables of nutritional allowances, or recommended intakes of nutrients, take into account such considerations. Many are available, drawn up by national and international committees. The nutritional allowances used in Britain since 1950 have been those recommended by the Committee on Nutrition of the British Medical Association. During the intervening years knowledge has accumulated that has made a review of the position desirable.

PURPOSE AND USE OF THE RECOMMENDATIONS

3. *The recommended intakes for nutrients* are defined as the amounts sufficient or more than sufficient for the nutritional needs of practically all healthy persons in a population. They do not cover any additional needs arising from diseases, such as infections, disorders of the gastrointestinal tract or metabolic abnormalities. The intake recommended for any one nutrient presupposes that the requirements for energy and all other nutrients are fully met. There is no evidence to suggest that intakes in excess of the recommendations confer any benefit; indeed, for energy and certain nutrients, intakes in excess may be harmful.

4. *The recommendations for energy* differ in a fundamental respect from those for nutrients. Although the detailed mechanism for the control of energy intake is not fully understood, an important factor is the level of energy expenditure; intake balances expenditure if the body is neither gaining nor losing weight. The recommended intake for energy is equated with the estimated average requirement, and therefore does not refer to individuals but only to groups.

5. The recommendations can be met by widely varying combinations of foods commonly consumed in the UK, and intakes of nutrients for which detailed recommendations are not given are then almost certainly sufficient. Expression of the recommendations on a daily basis does not imply that each must be met in full every day; the body can store any nutrient in sufficient quantity to last for at least a few days, and thus can accommodate irregular intakes.

The application of the recommendations

6. The recommendations may be used as guides for caterers and dietitians when planning diets for groups of healthy individuals. They may also be used in the evaluation of surveys of food consumption, and so in the identification of potential nutritional problems which merit further investigation. By themselves they cannot be used for the assessment of nutritional status, but are a useful adjunct to clinical and other studies.

7. The recommended intakes relate to the amounts of foods actually eaten. But food supplies may be measured on the plate, in the kitchen or larder, at the retail level in the shop or with wholesale distributors. In all these places there is likely to be wastage; also some specific nutrients may be lost during preparation or storage of foods. When interpreting the results of dietary surveys or planning nutritionally adequate diets, adjustments have to be made for these factors.

8. In a healthy community where there is no economic bar to obtaining palatable diets, appetite determines the distribution of energy intakes roughly in accordance with the varied needs of the individuals in a group. Therefore, provided the average observed energy intake is equal to the recommended intake for the group, and many people are not obtaining more than their requirements, few are likely to obtain less than they need, even though about half the individuals must of necessity obtain less energy than the average. If the average intake is appreciably greater than that recommended then, unless levels of activity have been underestimated, several are obtaining superfluous energy and are likely to become obese. Conversely, if the average intake is less than that recommended then, unless activity has been overestimated, undernutrition is present and some individuals will lose weight, or reduce their activity, or do both.

9. For nutrients, however, distribution of intake may be quite unrelated to distribution of need. The recommended intakes, which are judged to be sufficient for practically all individual members of a population, must of necessity be in excess of the requirements of most of them. If an individual is taking more of a nutrient than the recommended intake, he is almost certainly obtaining more than he requires; but if the average intake of a group is greater than the recommendation one cannot be sure that there is no malnutrition because of uncertainty about the distribution of intakes within the group. Equally, it is not legitimate to deduce the presence of malnutrition in a population merely on the basis of the results of a survey in which the average intake of a nutrient is less than the recommendation. But malnutrition is more likely to be present the further average intakes fall below the recommendations.

The provisional nature of the recommendations

10. Recommendations for intakes of nutrients can only be made by the exercise of judgment on limited data; in consequence they can only be provisional and subject to future revision in the light of new knowledge or change of circumstances.

11. In drawing up our recommendations we have made much use of the report of the Committee on Nutrition of the British Medical Association (BMA, 1950); reports of a Committee of the Food and Agriculture Organization on Calorie Requirements (FAO, 1957), and of Joint Expert Groups of the Food and Agriculture Organization and the World Health Organization on Protein Requirements (FAO/WHO, 1965), on Calcium Requirements (FAO/WHO, 1962), and on Requirements of Vitamin A, Thiamine, Riboflavine and Niacin (FAO/WHO, 1967); and of the reports on Recommended Dietary Allowances of the Food and Nutrition Board of the United States National Research Council (NRC, 1964, 1968).

12. Table 1 sets out our recommendations; we believe these to be sensible and practicable for the UK in 1969.

TABLE 1
Recommended Daily Intakes of Energy and Nutrients for the UK

(a) Age range	Occupational category	(c) Body weight kg	(d) Energy kcal	(d) Energy MJ	(f) Protein g	(g) Thiamine mg	Riboflavine mg	Nicotinic acid (h) mg equivalents	Ascorbic acid mg	Vitamin A (i) µg retinol equivalents	(j) Vitamin D µg cholecalciferol	Calcium mg	Iron mg
BOYS AND GIRLS												(l)	(l)
0 up to 1 year (b)		7.3	800	3.3	20	0.3	0.4	5	15	450	10	600	6
1 up to 2 years		11.4	1200	5.0	30	0.5	0.6	7	20	300	10	500	7
2 up to 3 years		13.5	1400	5.9	35	0.6	0.7	8	20	300	10	500	7
3 up to 5 years		16.5	1600	6.7	40	0.6	0.8	9	20	300	10	500	8
5 up to 7 years		20.5	1800	7.5	45	0.7	0.9	10	20	300	2.5	500	8
7 up to 9 years		25.1	2100	8.8	53	0.8	1.0	11	20	400	2.5	500	10
BOYS													
9 up to 12 years		31.9	2500	10.5	63	1.0	1.2	14	25	575	2.5	700	13
12 up to 15 years		45.5	2800	11.7	70	1.1	1.4	16	25	725	2.5	700	14
15 up to 18 years		61.0	3000	12.6	75	1.2	1.7	19	30	750	2.5	600	15
GIRLS													
9 up to 12 years		33.0	2300	9.6	58	0.9	1.2	13	25	575	2.5	700	13
12 up to 15 years		48.6	2300	9.6	58	0.9	1.4	16	25	725	2.5	700	14
15 up to 18 years		56.1	2300	9.6	58	0.9	1.4	16	30	750	2.5	600	15
MEN													
18 up to 35 years	Sedentary	65	2700	11.3	68	1.1	1.7	18	30	750	2.5	500	10
	Moderately active		3000	12.6	75	1.2	1.7	18	30	750	2.5	500	10
	Very active		3600	15.1	90	1.4	1.7	18	30	750	2.5	500	10
35 up to 65 years	Sedentary	65	2600	10.9	65	1.0	1.7	18	30	750	2.5	500	10
	Moderately active		2900	12.1	73	1.2	1.7	18	30	750	2.5	500	10
	Very active		3600	15.1	90	1.4	1.7	18	30	750	2.5	500	10
65 up to 75 years	} Assuming a sedentary life	63	2350	9.8	59	0.9	1.7	18	30	750	2.5	500	10
75 and over		63	2100	8.8	53	0.8	1.7	18	30	750	2.5	500	10
WOMEN													
18 up to 55 years	Most occupations	55	2200	9.2	55	0.9	1.3	15	30	750	2.5	500	12
	Very active		2500	10.5	63	1.0	1.3	15	30	750	2.5	500	12
55 up to 75 years	} Assuming a sedentary life	53	2050	8.6	51	0.8	1.3	15	30	750	2.5	500	10
75 and over		53	1900	8.0	48	0.7	1.3	15	30	750	2.5	500	10
Pregnancy, 2nd and 3rd trimester			2400	10.0	60	1.0	1.6	18	60	750	(k) 10	(m) 1200	15
Lactation			2700	11.3	68	1.1	1.8	21	60	1200	10	1200	15

Footnotes to Table 1

(a) The ages are from one birthday to another: e.g. 9 up to 12 is from the 9th up to, but not including, the 12th birthday. The figures in the Table in general refer to the mid-point of the ranges, though those for the range 18 up to 35 refer to the age 25 years, and for the range 18 up to 55, to 35 years of age.

(b) Average figures relating to the first year of life. Energy and minimum protein requirements for the four trimesters are given in Tables 2 and 3 respectively.

(c) The body weights of children and adolescents are averages and relate to London in 1965. (Taken from Tanner, Whitehouse & Takaishi, 1966; Tables IV A and IV B, 50th centile). The body weights of adults do not represent average values; they are those of the FAO (1957) reference man and woman, with a nominal reduction for the elderly.

(d) Average requirements relating to groups of individuals.

(e) Megajoules (10⁶ joules). Calculated from the relation 1 kilocalorie = 4·186 kilojoules, and rounded to 1 decimal place.

(f) Recommended intakes calculated as providing 10 per cent of energy requirements (see paragraph 64). Minimum protein requirements given in Table 3.

(g) The figures, calculated from energy requirements and the recommended intake of thiamine of 0·4 mg/1000 kcal, relate to groups of individuals.

(h) 1 nicotinic acid equivalent = 1 mg available nicotinic acid or 60 mg tryptophan.

(i) 1 retinol equivalent = 1 µg retinol or 6 µg β-carotene or 12 µg other biologically active carotenoids.

(j) No dietary source may be necessary for those adequately exposed to sunlight, but the requirement for the housebound may be greater than that recommended.

4

ENERGY

13. The body requires a source of energy to maintain the normal processes of life and to meet the demands of activity and growth. The unit of energy conventionally used by nutritionists is the kilocalorie (kcal.) However, it has been proposed that the joule should be used instead and for this reason in Tables 1 and 2 recommended intakes are given in both kilocalories and megajoules (1000 kcal=4.186 x 10^6 joules or 4.186 MJ).

14. Energy intake is defined as the sum of the metabolizable energy provided by the available carbohydrate, fat, protein and alcohol in the food ingested. Available carbohydrate is defined as the sum of the glucose, fructose, sucrose, maltose, lactose, dextrins and starches in the diet. In calculating the energy value of a diet the contributions, if any, from other carbohydrates e.g. cellulose, and from organic acids are ignored.

15. The procedure for calculating the metabolizable energy from the chemical composition of the diet is by the application of the appropriate energy conversion factors to the amounts of the energy-providing constituents in the diet. The choice of energy conversion factors is a subject of research and some controversy. In 'The Composition of Foods' (McCance & Widdowson, 1967) the factors used are: protein (total nitrogen times 5.7 for cereals, 6.38 for milk and 6.25 for all other foods) 4.1 kcal/g; fat 9.3 kcal/g; available carbohydrate, expressed as monosaccharides, 3.75 kcal/g; alcohol 7.0 kcal/g. These factors do not allow for losses of fat in the faeces; an allowance for this is made by the Ministry of Health and the Ministry of Agriculture, Fisheries and Food in calculating the results of individual dietary and national surveys, and the simpler factors used are 4.0, 9.0, 3.75 and 7.0 kcal/g of protein, fat, carbohydrate (as monosaccharides) and alcohol respectively. In practice, with usual UK diets, there is little difference between the total energy content of the diet as calculated by the two sets of factors.

16. Our recommendations for energy intake are based on values for energy expenditure or intake by samples of the UK population (Harries, Hobson & Hollingsworth, 1962; Durnin & Passmore, 1967). The recommended intakes are given in Tables 1 and 2. The weights for the age groups are based on measurements made in London by Tanner, Whitehouse & Takaishi (1966).

The Requirements of Adults

17. These are determined by the size and age of the individual and by the degree of physical activity.

The effect of body size

18. In the performance of standard tasks, body weight is an important determinant of an individual's energy expenditure; for instance, the energy cost of walking, in which most of the work is done by raising the centre of gravity at each step, is directly proportional to body weight.

19. However, an individual's total daily energy expenditure is not closely related to body weight. Durnin has examined the correlation between body weight and daily energy expenditure and found correlation coefficients no higher than 0.4. This lack of a close relation between body weight and daily energy

5

expenditure suggests that heavy people are less active than light. Indeed there is evidence that fat people are less physically active than lean individuals (Mayer & Bullen, 1964; Durnin, 1966). In calculating the energy needs of groups of adults in the UK the figures given in Table 1 may be used without correction for weight.

20. Energy requirements have frequently been related to surface area. There is now much evidence that the correlation of surface area with energy expenditure is no closer than that of body weight (Miller, 1968).

The effect of activity

21. For most men employed in an urban society the day is divided into three parts, each of about 8 hours. One part is spent in bed and asleep, one at work, including travelling to work, and the third in non-occupational activities which include recreations.

22. The energy expenditure in bed and asleep is the resting metabolism, which is related to body size, but otherwise varies little; for a 65 kg man it is about 500 kcal/8 hr (Appendix 1). At work the energy expenditure is determined mainly by the occupation and relatively little by the individual. The energy expenditure in non-occupational activities is determined by the individual and not by his occupation, as discussed in paragraph 26.

23. The BMA (1950) used an elaborate series of six grades for men with allowances ranging from 2250 to 5000 kcal/day according to occupational activity, and five grades for women ranging from 2000 to 3750 kcal/day. The higher levels of activity are observed rarely nowadays and extremely high levels of energy expenditure are only maintained for short periods of time. We have reduced the number of groups to three for men and two for women.

24. Within the same nominal occupation, there is wide variation in the nature of the work which is carried out, and for this reason guidance as to the classification of occupational activity can only be given in a broad sense. In Table 1 men are divided into sedentary, moderately active and very active groups with recommended intakes of 2700, 3000 and 3600 kcal/day respectively. A rough guide for assessing the needs of men is as follows:

Sedentary: Office workers (all clerical tasks), drivers, pilots, teachers, journalists, clergy, doctors, lawyers, architects and shop workers.

Moderately active: Virtually all engaged in light industry and assembly plants; railway workers, postmen, joiners, slaters, plumbers and bus conductors; most farm workers and builders' labourers.

Very active: Coal miners, steel workers, dockers, forestry workers and army recruits; some farm workers, builders' labourers and unskilled labourers.

25. The energy requirement for many occupations depends on the amount of mechanical power available. Thus farmers and workers in the building industry may often do heavy work, but on a modern farm or building site the men are usually no more than moderately active. Heavy work may be carried out for only short periods throughout the day and, unless these add up to over 60 minutes, the occupation should be classified as only moderately active. Eight hours of sedentary work involves an energy expenditure of about 900 kcal, of moderately active work about 1200 kcal and of heavy work about 1800 kcal.

26. Individual energy expenditure may depend as much on variations in recreational and non-occupational activities as on occupation. This expenditure commonly ranges from as low as 800 to about 1800 kcal in the course of the day. There is no evidence that the recreational activities of sedentary and heavy workers differ significantly: not a few heavy workers are keen participants in sport and many clerks are television addicts. Because we are recommending intakes for groups and not individuals and the variation in non-occupational energy expenditure is likely to be similar in groups within different occupations, it is feasible to recommend average intakes of energy for different categories of occupation as in paragraph 24.

27. The energy expenditure for each category of occupation can be thought of as distributed in the following way:

Occupation:	Sedentary	Moderately active	Very active
Energy expenditure			
in bed (kcal/8 hr)	500	500	500
at work (kcal/8 hr)	900	1200	1800
non-occupational (kcal/8 hr)	800–1800	800–1800	800–1800
Energy requirement from			
food (kcal/24 hr)	2200–3200	2500–3500	3100–4100
Recommended intake for			
a group (kcal/24 hr)	2700	3000	3600

28. For most groups of women the daily recommended intake is 2200 kcal. Of this, an average of about 880 kcal is required for 8 hours of occupational activity in the home, an office or light industry, about 900 kcal for 8 hours of non-occupational activity, and 420 kcal for 8 hours in bed. For those whose work or recreation demands significantly more than average physical activity, an extra 300 kcal is added to give a total of 2500 kcal/day (Table 1).

29. These recommendations are lower than those of FAO (1957). Many surveys have shown that in the UK both occupational and non-occupational energy expenditure is less than that of the FAO reference man and woman. However, the USA recommended dietary intakes (NRC, 1968) are even lower than ours, being 2800 kcal for young men and 2000 kcal for young women. These figures probably correspond closely to average rates of energy expenditure in the USA. We would not recommend further reduction to the USA level at the present time. Such a reduction may be necessary in the future if increased mechanization and better organization of industry results in diminished energy expenditure at work, unless this is compensated for by increased participation in active recreations. As many of the degenerative diseases of middle age arise in part as a result of inactivity, it would be better if such compensation did take place.

The effect of age

30. With increasing age there is a gradual decline in the metabolism at rest and therefore a reduced need for energy in the diet. A relatively greater reduction results from the gradual slowing down of the individual and the diminishing physical activity. The recommendations given in Table 1 for energy intakes

for the middle aged, the elderly and the very old are based on our judgement of the rates at which most people slow down. Surveys of energy expenditure and energy intake in relation to age are discussed by Durnin & Passmore (1967).

31. In Table 1 the range for men over 35 has been extended to 65 so that the upper limit now corresponds with the normal age of retirement for men, at which age it was considered that a change in physical activity probably occurs. Women aged 18–55 have been classified together.

32. It should be emphasized that not a few people retain their active habits of life until they are 75 or even older. They need more energy in their diet than the figures given in Table 1. Perhaps a larger number lose their active habits earlier in life. If they continue to eat as formerly, then inevitably they become obese.

The Requirements of Infants, Children and Adolescents

Infants

33. Energy requirements, when related to body weight, fall progressively from birth. The values are about 100 kcal/kg daily between the ages of 6 months and 1 year (Bransby & Fothergill, 1954; Ministry of Health, 1968). There is a poor correlation between energy intake and body weight, and therefore daily recommended intakes are also given in Table 2 for the four trimesters in the first year of life. An average value for the year as a whole is given in Table 1. The daily output of breast milk provides similar amounts of energy to those recommended for early infancy.

TABLE 2

Recommended daily intakes of energy for infants

Age range	Body weight kg	kcal/kg	kcal	MJ
Birth up to 3 months	4·6	120	550	2·3
3 up to 6 months	6·6	115	760	3·2
6 up to 9 months	8·3	110	910	3·8
9 up to 12 months	9·5	105	1000	4·2

Children and adolescents

34. The differences in body weight and physical activity between the second and third years of life make it desirable to recommend separately for these two years. A break is made at age five to coincide with the start of primary schooling, which may well be associated with a change in activity. The only comprehensive data are from a pre-war survey of energy intake made by Widdowson (1947). Bransby & Fothergill (1954) and the Ministry of Health (1968) provide values for some younger children which confirm that Widdowson's data are still applicable today.

35. For boys between 9 and 18, the values given in Table 1 are based on Widdowson (1947) and, where appropriate, Fowke (1945) and Durnin & Lonergan (1968). The values for girls between 9 and 18 were chosen in a similar

fashion; values recommended for the oldest range (15–18) are not raised, as they are for the boys, because of the high prevalence of obesity amongst girls of this age.

The Requirements during Pregnancy and Lactation

Pregnancy

36. Requirements are raised during pregnancy by the needs of the growing fetus and by adjustments to the metabolism and the body composition of the mother. Experimental observations and calculations suggest that, for a healthy woman who gains about 12·5 kg body weight, the requirement is about 80,000 kcal for the whole of pregnancy (FAO, 1957; Hytten & Leitch, 1964). This is additional to the needs of a non-pregnant woman, with a similar level of physical activity; a high proportion of it is accounted for by storage of maternal body fat.

37. In Western civilization it is not necessary to meet this extra energy requirement of pregnancy in full, because pregnancy usually reduces physical activity. There are no data from which the probable extent of such compensation can be estimated. FAO (1957) thought that the physiological requirement might be halved, and that an additional allowance of 40,000 kcal per pregnancy would be satisfactory.

38. Commonly in pregnancy food intake is slightly reduced during the first trimester, possibly due to nausea. Early in the second trimester a surge of appetite compensates for the previous reduction; and thereafter food intake is slightly decreased. Variations between individuals and from stage to stage in each individual are large, and many women are advised by their doctors to curb their appetites in order to restrict the weight gained.

39. From the evidence at our disposal, an additional intake of 200 kcal/day during the second and third trimester (36,000 kcal/pregnancy) may be regarded as realistic in practice and physiologically adequate.

Lactation

40. FAO (1957) and the NRC (1968) recommend an additional allowance of 1000 kcal/day during lactation. The estimate is based on an assumed milk production of 850 ml/day (equivalent to about 600 kcal), the energy in food being converted to energy in milk with an efficiency of about 60 per cent.

41. An additional allowance of 1000 kcal implies that the total energy intake of the average lactating woman exceeds 3000 kcal/day. FAO comment that: "In practice, some women find that an increase of calorie intake of 1000 calories daily is not easily achieved and an increase of 800 kcal may be a more realistic estimate".

42. Hytten & Thomson (1961) provide evidence that the efficiency of human milk production is about 80 per cent, not 60 per cent as previously thought, and that the cost of milk production is subsidized to some extent by utilizing reserves of body fat which have been laid down during pregnancy. On this basis, the fact that many lactating women slowly lose weight is not evidence of dietary insufficiency, but of the readjustment of fat depots at the end of a reproductive cycle.

9

43. There seems to be little doubt that healthy women in the UK do not increase their food intake by nearly as much as 1000 kcal/day, and that the physiological adjustments of pregnancy include the laying down of extra reserves of maternal fat. Thus an additional daily intake during lactation of 500 kcal seems adequate, both in relation to physiological needs and to the food habits of lactating women in the UK. This figure is less than the recommended intake for infants because, if a mother has laid down about 4 kg of fat during pregnancy (Hytten & Leitch, 1964), which she loses during lactation, this provides some 36,000 kcal toward the cost of the milk supply.

PROTEIN

44. Dietary proteins are split during digestion into their constituent amino acids, which are required to replace the tissues broken down during the normal processes of living and to form new tissue for growth. A particular difficulty arises because protein supplies both energy and nutrients. When the intake of food is inadequate to meet the energy demands of the tissues, amino acids which might otherwise be used for the synthesis of body protein are oxidized instead to provide energy; protein requirements cannot then be met by increasing the proportion of protein in the diet, but only by increasing the total energy intake.

Protein quality

45. Proteins in the diet vary in their usefulness to the body, depending on the extent to which they contain the essential amino acids—those that cannot be synthesized within the body—in the proportions required for making new tissue. A mixture of proteins may be more useful for this purpose than a single protein, because a deficiency of an amino acid in one protein may be made up by a high proportion of that amino acid in another. In assessing the value to the body of a protein or a mixture of proteins, it is convenient to use a comparison with a hypothetical protein that would be completely incorporated without waste into the body tissues. Such a protein, a "reference protein", is said to have a net protein utilization (NPU) of 100. If x grams of reference protein are needed, $2x$ grams of a protein that is only 50 per cent utilized and $1.5x$ grams of one 67 per cent utilized are required.

46. There are other factors besides the amino acid composition and the energy intake in the diet that may affect the value of a dietary protein (Miller & Payne, 1961); for example, it also depends on the proportion of the total energy supplied by protein, and on food processing, during which the amino acids may be destroyed or made unavailable. The mixed proteins of diets eaten in the UK have a NPU of about 70 per cent (Greaves & Tan, 1966a).

47. Protein is assessed quantitatively in the diet from estimations of its nitrogen content. The proportion of nitrogen in different proteins varies from about 15·7 to 19 per cent, but it is customary to take it as 16 per cent and to use the factor of 6·25 (100/16) to convert nitrogen to protein.

The Minimum Requirements for Nitrogen

48. Studies of nitrogen balance and the calculation of the additional nitrogen needed for growth, pregnancy and lactation provide sufficient information for estimating minimum requirements.

Nitrogen balance

49. Nitrogen losses from the body in the urine and faeces can be easily measured. There are relatively small losses in the sweat and in the growth of hair, nails and skin for which an allowance can be made. Nitrogen in the urine results from the breakdown of protein in the normal metabolic processes of the body; the amount depends on the protein content of the diet, but even when the diet contains no protein, there is always a basal or endogenous urinary loss of

11

nitrogen. The faeces contain nitrogen derived from protein of the digestive enzymes and shed epithelial cells of the intestinal tract, as well as from the diet.

50. An adult man taking in his diet sufficient or more than sufficient nitrogen for his protein needs loses an amount exactly equal to his intake. Such a person is said to be in nitrogen equilibrium. If the intake falls below the body's needs, the man is in negative nitrogen balance, since the losses are greater than his intake. By experiment one can find the least amount of dietary protein that produces this overall state of nitrogen equilibrium, and this represents the minimum needs for maintenance for the adult. In this situation the sum of the amounts lost also gives the nitrogen requirement for maintenance and therefore provides an estimate of the minimum amount needed to be made available from the food.

Requirement for maintenance

51. To calculate requirements for maintenance of people of different ages the sum of the nitrogen losses must in some way be related to body size. Nitrogen metabolism depends on cell mass (Appendix 1) and is only indirectly related to body weight and other factors such as surface area. Both nitrogen metabolism and cell mass are closely related to the resting energy metabolism (basal metabolic rate) which can be measured, and figures are available for various ages (Appendix 1). If the resting metabolism is taken into account, the amount of metabolic nitrogen lost can be derived for people of different ages and sex.

52. The daily nitrogen requirements for maintenance are 2·65 mg N/basal kcal made up in the following way.

(a) Endogenous urinary loss: the minimum daily loss in the urine due to breakdown of protein in the body is 2·0 mg N/kcal (FAO/WHO, 1965).

(b) Metabolic faecal loss: minimum daily loss in the faeces is taken as 0·57 mg N/kcal. This is the average of the range of values given by FAO/WHO (1965); they used a figure equivalent to 0·9 mg, which is at the higher end of the range. The NRC (1964, 1968) took 0·4 mg.

(c) Daily skin losses; these are taken as 0·08 mg N/kcal, a value derived from the results of Sirbu, Margen & Calloway (1967). FAO/WHO (1965) took a much higher figure equivalent to 0·8 mg N. These high values however are not in accord with the results of Darke (1960) or the recent work of Ashworth & Harrower (1967).

Special requirements

53. Children and pregnant and lactating women all need more nitrogen than that required for maintenance. Nitrogen must be retained in the body for the growth of the child, or of the fetus and maternal tissues, and for the secretion of milk.

54. *Requirement for growth.* The nitrogen content of the tissue laid down during growth is calculated from the weight increment and the nitrogen concentration of the body. Weight increments of children at different ages are taken from Tanner, Whitehouse & Takaishi (1966). The nitrogen concentration in the whole body is taken as 1·83 per cent at birth, increasing to 2·34 per cent

at the age of one year (Fomon, 1967). Values at ages between one year and 4 years, when adult proportions have been reached, are obtained by interpolation between this figure and 2·9 per cent, the figure based on the results of whole body analyses (Widdowson & Dickerson, 1964).

55. *Requirements for pregnancy and lactation.* The protein content of the products of conception and of the increased weight of the maternal reproductive tissues has been taken as 950 g (FAO/WHO, 1965), which is met by an increase of 0·54 g in the daily intake of nitrogen. An average daily milk output of 850 ml has been assumed (FAO/WHO, 1965), with an average protein content of 1·2 per cent. Thus, the total daily nitrogen output in the milk is 1·6 g which needs to be replaced by increasing the dietary intake.

Individual variation

56. It is difficult to make allowances for all the factors that affect requirements, such as variations between individuals and increases due to everyday stresses. However, the variation between individuals can be derived from figures published for several groups of adults who were presumably subject to normal stresses (Appendix 2). By increasing the minimum requirements for nitrogen by 20 per cent, the requirements of the great majority of people are covered.

The Minimum Requirements for Protein

57. For the calculation of protein requirements, the nitrogen requirements for maintenance are first related to the resting metabolism for the appropriate age and sex; where necessary the supplementary nitrogen needed for growth, pregnancy or lactation is added. The total is converted to protein by multiplying by 6·25; a factor of 100/70 allows for the efficiency of utilization of the dietary protein (paragraph 46), and an addition of 20 per cent covers the individual variation.

58. *Example of calculation.* A group of boys aged 4 to 6 years grow at an average rate of 5·3 g/day (Tanner, Whitehouse & Takaishi, 1966). Their resting metabolism would be 850 kcal/24 hr (Appendix 1) and their bodies would contain 2·9 per cent N (paragraph 54).

Thus,

Nitrogen for maintenance $= \dfrac{850 \times 2·65}{1000} = 2·25$ g/day

Nitrogen for growth $= \dfrac{5·3 \times 2·9}{100} = 0·15$ g/day

Total nitrogen requirements $= 2·40$ g/day

Protein requirement $= 2·40 \times 6·25 = 15·0$ g/day

Provision for efficiency of utilization $= 15·0 \times \dfrac{100}{70} = 21·4$ g/day

Provision for individual variation $= 21·4 + 20\% = 25·3$ g/day

Therefore the minimum requirement for protein for boys aged 4 to 6 years is 25 g/day.

59. Minimum requirements for protein calculated in this way are given in Table 3. On this basis the requirement for the adult man weighing 65 kg is 45 g/day. For the adult woman the requirement is 38 g/day with an additional allowance of 6 g/day during pregnancy and 17 g/day for lactation. The Table also shows the percentage of the total energy requirement provided by these amounts of protein (Pcals %), taking the factor of 4 kcal/g protein (paragraph 15).

60. Persons taking the amounts set out in Table 3 of the type of protein provided by mixed diets in the UK (see paragraph 46) are unlikely to suffer from deficiency of protein. Several studies in which diets low in protein have been fed, some of them with vitamin supplements, provide evidence that these amounts are satisfactory for periods of weeks or even months. Fomon (1960) has done repeated metabolic balance studies and followed the growth of infants up to the age of 6 months on a milk mixture providing 1·03 g protein/100 ml, a content comparable to that of human milk. Nitrogen retention in these infants was similar to that in breast fed infants and their growth rate and serum protein concentration were normal. Later work (Fomon, 1967) has confirmed these rates of weight gain on various mixtures, and has shown no benefit in feeding young infants diets containing 20 per cent of the calories from cows milk protein. Chan & Waterlow (1966) have successfully treated infants recovering from protein deficiency with diets containing similar amounts of protein to those in Table 3.

61. In older age groups, Harper (1960) and James (1960) found nitrogen retention to be consistent with the demands of growth in children aged 6 to 9 years when fed on diets containing 18 to 22 g protein/day or about 4 per cent of energy from protein over a period of 48 days. Bricker, Shively, Smith, Mitchell & Hamilton (1949) maintained 9 young college women on intakes of 20 to 35 g protein/day for 10 weeks; the blood picture and performance tests were entirely satisfactory. The classical work of Chittenden (1905), not only on himself but on professional colleagues, soldiers and athletes over periods of 9 months to a year, showed that daily intakes of 40 to 50 g of protein were consistent with full health.

62. There is evidence therefore that these minimal amounts of protein maintain nitrogen balance and allow for normal growth in infants and children at least for limited periods. However, we cannot exclude the possiblity that some tissues may suffer preferentially while the overall nitrogen balance is apparently unaffected. The question of whether the minimum requirements are adequate to maintain health for a life-time can only be answered by long-term studies, which have not yet been made. A Working Party of the Ministry of Health in 1963 calculated minimum requirements using the same principle that we have used here and called these figures a lower limit of knowledge because they also recognized the limitations of the evidence. They considered the actual quantities of protein eaten by people in the UK as an upper limit of knowledge, and regarded the physiological requirements as falling between the two (Ministry of Health, 1964).

The Recommended Intake

63. Ordinary diets in the UK contain amounts of protein substantially greater than those in Table 3, the majority of people taking between 10 and 15 per cent

of their energy in the form of protein (Greaves & Hollingsworth, 1964). The fact that this relatively high proportion of protein has been eaten in the UK for generations suggests that this plays a part in making the diets acceptable, and there is no evidence that any harm results from such amounts. It cannot be emphasized too strongly that in the construction of diets attention must be paid to palatability as well as to nutrient content.

64. Diets containing protein at the level of the minimum requirement would be unlikely to be palatable; furthermore, the recommended intakes of some of the other nutrients such as riboflavine and nicotinic acid, and satisfactory amounts of other B vitamins often found in association with dietary protein, might not be provided. For these reasons we have increased the recommended intake of protein above the minimum requirement so that it approaches more closely known dietary habits. An arbitrary value of 10 per cent of the total energy requirement has been chosen for the recommended intake of protein since few diets in the UK provide less, and we can be confident that the reservations about the minimum requirement mentioned in paragraph 62 would not apply at this level. Amounts of protein calculated in this way, assuming that 1 g protein provides 4 kcal, are shown in Table 1.

65. *Summary.* First, we have calculated minimum requirements of protein of NPU 70 per cent which are set out in Table 3. These amounts, so long as requirements for other nutrients are satisfied, would be sufficient to prevent the appearance of protein deficiency disease. The table could be used in assessing the adequacy of the protein content of diets. Secondly, in accordance with dietary habits in the UK, recommended intakes that provide 10 per cent of the total energy requirements as protein are given in Table 1. It is this Table that should therefore be used for the planning and construction of diets.

TABLE 3
Minimum requirements for protein

Age range	Occupational category	Body weight	Energy requirement	Minimum requirement for protein (NPU 70%)	
		kg	kcal/day	g/day	P cals %
A	B	C	D	E	F
Infants					
Birth up to 3 months		4·6	550	13	9·5
3 up to 6 months		6·6	760	14	7·4
6 up to 9 months		8·3	910	15	6·6
9 up to 12 months		9·5	1000	16	6·4
Boys and Girls					
1 up to 2 years		11·4	1200	19	6·3
2 up to 3 years		13·5	1400	21	6·1
3 up to 5 years		16·5	1600	25	6·1
5 up to 7 years		20·5	1800	28	6·1
7 up to 9 years		25·1	2100	30	5·7
Boys					
9 up to 12 years		31·9	2500	36	5·8
12 up to 15 years		45·5	2800	46	6·6
15 up to 18 years		61·0	3000	50	6·7
Girls					
9 up to 12 years		33·0	2300	35	6·1
12 up to 15 years		48·6	2300	44	7·6
15 up to 18 years		56·1	2300	40	7·0
Men					
18 up to 35 years	Sedentary	65	2700	45	6·7
	Moderately active		3000	45	6·0
	Very active		3600	45	5·0
35 up to 65 years	Sedentary	65	2600	43	6·6
	Moderately active		2900	43	5·9
	Very active		3600	43	4·8
65 up to 75 years }	Assuming a	63	2350	39	6·6
75 and over }	sedentary life	63	2100	38	7·2
Women					
18 up to 55 years	Most occupations	55	2200	38	6·9
	Very active		2500	38	6·1
55 up to 75 years }	Assuming a	53	2050	36	7·0
75 and over }	sedentary life	53	1900	34	7·2
Pregnancy			2400	44	7·3
Lactation			2700	55	8·1

Notes: 1. *Columns A, B, C, D* as in Tables 1 and 2.
2. The amounts of protein given in *Column E* are sufficient to prevent the appearance of protein deficiency in most individuals, and may be used in assessing the adequacy of the protein content of diets.
3. *Column F* calculated as $\frac{E \times 4}{D} \times 100$.

VITAMINS

66. The vitamins are organic substances which the body requires in relatively small amounts for its metabolism, but which it cannot make for itself, at least in sufficient quantity. Historically the vitamins have been classified as being soluble either in water (the B vitamins and vitamin C) or in fat solvents, and they are treated below in this order. However, this classification does not imply that they are either chemically or functionally related. The B vitamins have been shown to act as specific cofactors in enzyme systems, but the physiological action of the other vitamins is not in general so well understood.

Thiamine (Vitamin B₁)

67. Thiamine in its biologically active form of thiamine pyrophosphate (cocarboxylase) functions as a coenzyme in the decarboxylation of pyruvic and α-ketoglutaric acids, and in the direct oxidation of glucose to yield pentoses (transketolase system). Thiamine deficiency leads to beriberi, which has been a major disease in many parts of the world. The disease is rare in the UK and there is no evidence that any section of the population, except some chronic alcoholics, suffer from thiamine deficiency.

Requirements

68. Animal experiments have shown that the rate of thiamine utilization depends on the amount of carbohydrate metabolized, and epidemiological studies in man also indicate that thiamine requirements are closely related to carbohydrate intake. However, little precision is lost if they are related to the total energy intake and it is now the general practice to express requirements for thiamine per 1000 kcal ingested (but see paragraph 71). Increased physical activity, pregnancy and lactation increase thiamine requirements because of the greater energy need; but when expressed per 1000 kcal the requirement for thiamine is constant, and this relationship does not vary in such circumstances or with age.

69. Thiamine requirements have been estimated by measuring the amount of the vitamin or its metabolites excreted in the urine following an oral dose, or by the identification of abnormalities in carbohydrate metabolism with respect to thiamine intake. Thiamine intakes ranging from 0·2 to 0·5 mg/1000 kcal have been reported to satisfy minimum requirements, but usually 0·2 mg/1000 kcal is sufficient. The level required to give tissue saturation is accepted as being 0·3 to 0·35 mg/1000 kcal, any excess being excreted. From this evidence FAO/WHO (1967) suggested an average thiamine requirement of 0·33 mg/1000 kcal.

Recommended intake

70. FAO/WHO (1967) made an allowance for individual variation in thiamine requirements on the basis of the variation in resting energy expenditure, for which the standard deviation has been estimated to be about 10 per cent of the mean. The average requirement was increased by 20 per cent to give a recommended intake of 0·4 mg thiamine/1000 kcal. In Great Britain in 1966 the average thiamine intake was 0·52 mg/1000 kcal (Ministry of Agriculture, Fisheries and Food, 1968). We accept the FAO/WHO report and recommend for thiamine an intake of 0·4 mg/1000 kcal.

71. The recommended intake has been applied in Table 1 to the average energy requirements for different categories of people, and the resulting figures thus relate to groups and not to individuals. Because of the considerations mentioned in paragraph 68, thiamine requirements are reduced in persons whose carbohydrate intake contributes substantially less to the energy value of the diet than the 40 to 50 per cent usual in the UK.

Availability and stability

72. Thiamine is widely distributed in foods and in general is available to man. Freshwater fish, molluscs and certain crustaceans contain enzymes (thiaminases) which destroy the vitamin. These enzymes are destroyed by heating and have not been reported to cause human thiamine deficiency in the UK.

73. Thiamine is soluble in water, sensitive to oxidation and unstable in foods subjected to high temperatures. It is destroyed rapidly by heat in neutral or alkaline solutions and large amounts may be lost during cooking and in the processing of foods. Roasting and stewing of meat may reduce the thiamine content by 30 to 50 per cent and vegetables may lose 25 to 40 per cent on cooking. These losses are increased by the use of bicarbonate of soda in cooking or the treatment of foods with sulphite. Prolonged storage of most foods may result in a significant loss of thiamine, the degree of loss depending upon conditions such as pH and temperature. Frozen foods stored at −18°C show little loss of the vitamin for periods of up to 1 year.

Riboflavine

74. Riboflavine forms the prosthetic group of flavoproteins, which are involved in hydrogen transport systems in the respiratory chain. Deficiency of riboflavine produces lesions in mucous membranes, most easily seen in the tongue, lips and cornea.

Method of expressing riboflavine requirements

75. Riboflavine requirements are related to the level of energy intake by FAO/WHO (1967). However, the requirement does not alter with varying activity and appears to be related more closely with endogenous protein utilization, metabolic body size or cell mass. The various methods of expression give similar values at ordinary intake levels and only deviate when the energy requirements are especially high or below 2000 kcal. Cell mass is correlated closely with resting metabolism, which is easily measured (Appendix 1), and we have used an expression relating requirements to resting metabolism for deriving our recommendations.

Requirements

76. The riboflavine requirements were reviewed by Bro-Rasmussen (1958) and again by FAO/WHO (1967). Riboflavine intakes below 0·3 mg/1000 kcal have been associated with clinical signs of deficiency. A sharp rise in riboflavine excretion occurs when the daily intake exceeds 0·44 mg/1000 kcal. This level probably represents tissue "saturation". There is no evidence, however, that people with tissue saturation are more healthy than those on levels which just prevent clinical signs of deficiency. Measurement of riboflavine in the urine shows that intakes below 1·1 mg/day cannot maintain a tissue reserve in adult males.

77. There is no evidence in human beings that the requirement of riboflavine is influenced by the carbohydrate/fat ratio, although such evidence exists in some animal species. The requirement is not apparently related to the increase in energy during physical activity, nor to climate.

Recommended intake

78. FAO/WHO (1967) have accepted 0·44 mg/1000 kcal as the average riboflavine requirement. Making allowance for individual variation they advised 0·55 mg/1000 kcal for the recommended intake, a figure similar to that used by many other countries and which we accept as the basis of our recommendations.

79. On this basis the recommended intake of riboflavine for an adult male weighing 65 kg and requiring 3000 kcal is 1·7 mg/day, equivalent to 0·07 mg/kg$^{0.75}$ or 1 mg/1000 resting kcal. For calculating the recommended intakes for the different categories of persons given in Table 1, the latter expression has been used together with values of resting metabolism given in Appendix 1. Thus the recommended intake for women is 1·3 mg/day.

80. *The elderly.* Because resting metabolism and energy intakes decrease with age the recommended intake of riboflavine would be reduced if either of these parameters were used for the elderly. However, we know of no evidence that the requirements of the elderly for riboflavine are less than those of younger adults, and we recommend that intakes of riboflavine should not fall with increasing age (Table 1).

81. *Pregnancy and lactation.* Increased requirements during the latter stages of pregnancy may be estimated as 0·3 mg/day. The recommended intake for pregnant women thus becomes 1·6 mg/day. About 0·3 mg to 0·5 mg riboflavine are secreted daily in breast milk, and we recommend a daily intake of 1·8 mg during lactation.

Sources and stability

82. Riboflavine is soluble in water and is widely distributed in all leafy vegetables, in the flesh of animals and fish and in milk. It may be destroyed when food is left exposed to sunlight (e.g. milk in bottles). Losses also occur in the preparation and cooking of foods, but the overall loss in food preparation is small and much less than the corresponding losses of thiamine and ascorbic acid.

Nicotinic Acid

83. Nicotinic acid (sometimes called niacin) is incorporated into the pyridine nucleotide coenzymes, which function as cofactors for many enzyme reactions involved in electron transfer. Deficiency of nicotinic acid results in pellagra.

84. Nicotinic acid is widely distributed, particularly in animal foods and legumes. In cereals it is present in a bound form and is largely unavailable. The amino acid tryptophan is converted to nicotinic acid in the body and is therefore an important source of the vitamin. It is not known how much the conversion of tryptophan to nicotinic acid is affected when tryptophan is the limiting factor in the diet.

Units

85. Nicotinic acid requirements have hitherto been expressed in mg/1000 kcal. There is little evidence that this parameter is correct, and by analogy with riboflavine which has a similar function it is proposed to calculate the allowance in terms of cell mass, or more specifically, resting metabolism (paragraph 75). Since about 60 mg tryptophan produce 1 mg nicotinic acid, intake can be measured in nicotinic acid equivalents. One mg nicotinic acid equivalent is defined as being equal to 1 mg of available nicotinic acid or 60 mg of tryptophan.

Requirements

86. The minimum intake for the prevention of clinical deficiency in adults is 4·4 mg nicotinic acid equivalents/1000 kcal. However, depletion-repletion experiments, involving the determination of the urinary excretion of N′-methylnicotinamide with different dietary supplements, showed that at this level of intake biochemical abnormalities were present. FAO/WHO (1967) accepted that 5·5 mg nicotinic acid equivalents/1000 kcal, an intake at which no clinical signs were observed and at which some of the subjects showed an increase in urinary excretion of nicotinic acid metabolites, represented the average requirement.

87. No significant effect on the nicotinic acid requirement of nutrients other than tryptophan in the diet is known, except that diets deficient in protein may give rise to an amino acid imbalance and perhaps increase the requirement. There is no evidence that physical activity increases the requirement and this is an argument against relating requirements to energy intake.

Recommended intake

88. Allowing for individual variation FAO/WHO (1967) recommended a daily intake of 6·6 mg nicotinic acid equivalents/1000 kcal, which we accept as the basis of our recommendations. However, this figure was calculated from diets in which 20 to 40 per cent of the nicotinic acid was derived from cereals, which may be presumed to be unavailable (paragraph 90). This reduces the recommended intake to 6·1 mg nicotinic acid equivalents/1000 kcal, or 11·4 mg nicotinic acid equivalents/1000 resting kcal, which is used to calculate the figures in Table 1 (cf. paragraph 79). Thus, the daily recommended intake for the adult man is 18 mg nicotinic acid equivalents, and for the adult woman 15 mg nicotinic acid equivalents. As for riboflavine (paragraph 80) we do not recommend that the intake of nicotinic acid equivalents in adults should fall with increasing age, although cell mass and resting metabolism decrease.

89. *Pregnancy and lactation*. An increased intake of 3 mg nicotinic acid equivalents/day during pregnancy is recommended. During lactation 4 to 6 mg nicotinic acid equivalents/day are secreted in human milk; accordingly, an increase of 6 mg in the intake is recommended during lactation.

Availability and stability

90. Nicotinic acid from animal sources and legumes is present as free nicotinamide or nicotinamide adenine dinucleotides and is therefore available (Chaudhuri & Kodicek, 1949). In cereals, little or no free nicotinamide is present, the vitamin being bound as nicotinic acid in a complex molecule called "niacytin"

20

(Kodicek, 1962), and probably not released *in vivo* to any significant extent. Evidence for the unavailability of niacytin to humans is scarce (Clegg, 1963), but for practical purposes cereal products, unless fortified, should be discounted as a source of preformed nicotinic acid, although the tryptophan they contain does contribute to the vitamin intake. Nicotinic acid and nicotinamide are stable in the usual conditions of processing and food preparation, but could be lost during cooking due to their solubility in water.

Vitamin B_6

91. Vitamin B_6 is a collective term for pyridoxol, pyridoxal and pyridoxamine; the three forms are interconvertible in the body. Most of the functions of the vitamin are concerned with the metabolism of amino acids, and the dietary requirement is therefore related to the intake of protein. Deficiency diseases in animals due to lack of the vitamin can be readily produced. Very occasionally infants develop convulsions and other disturbances of the central nervous system which respond to treatment with doses of the vitamin far in excess of normal intakes. Such infants may be said to have an idiosyncrasy which increases their need for the vitamin. In adults, hypochromic anaemia occasionally arises which responds only to the vitamin. Most diets in this country provide 1 to 2 mg/day and this appears to be enough for most people.

Folic Acid and Vitamin B_{12}

92. Both these vitamins are involved in the synthesis of nucleoproteins. Deficiency causes megaloblastic anaemia. The terms folic acid and folate are commonly used as group names to refer to the various biologically active forms of pteroylglutamic acid (PGA), although folic acid is sometimes used for PGA itself. Naturally occurring folate is chiefly in the form of formyl or methyl derivatives of tetrahydrofolic acid (reduced PGA), conjugated with additional glutamic acid residues, known as polyglutamates. The vitamin is widely distributed in foods; rich sources are yeast, liver, spinach and lettuce. There is doubt about the relative potencies for man of the different natural forms, but probably most dietary polyglutamates can be utilized, at least to some extent.

93. Studies on man suggest that the requirement, in terms of pure PGA, is about 50 to 100 μg/day, although in pregnancy it may be 400 μg or more. Measurement of activity in food is done mostly by microbiological assay, and estimates of activity vary widely, according to the choice of organism and the conditions of assay. Thus mixed diets have been estimated, by one method, to provide about 200 μg of folate daily, and by another method, over 600 μg (Butterworth, 1968). Folate activity may be reduced by cooking, especially by prolonged boiling in water, and by pH changes in the gastrointestinal tract.

94. Megaloblastic anaemia arising from folic acid deficiency occurs in this country under four circumstances:
    (i) failure to absorb the vitamin, which is a common complication of chronic disease of the small intestine;
    (ii) in pregnancy, where it is not common, but if it does occur is often severe; indeed, unless adequately treated it may be fatal, and for this reason during the last trimester of pregnancy a routine daily supple-

21

ment is frequently prescribed: a daily dose of 100 μg PGA is probably sufficient;

(iii) occasionally in infants, especially in the premature and those with infections; and

(iv) sometimes in old age, when due to apathy, ignorance or poor appetite, intakes may be low.

95. There have been many reports of low levels of folate in the serum or red blood cells of patients in mental hospitals and on admission to geriatric units. The low levels may be due to either a low dietary intake or poor absorption in the intestine. These findings emphasize the importance of ensuring that all old people and mental patients receive a good mixed diet.

96. Megaloblastic anaemia due to deficiency of vitamin B_{12} (cobalamin) is well recognized as arising secondary to a failure of absorption, when it is known as Addisonian pernicious anaemia. The vitamin is found only in foods of animal origin, but as little as 3 to 4 μg/day is sufficient. Dietary vitamin B_{12} deficiency is exceedingly rare in this country, though it has been reported occasionally in strict vegetarians or vegans, who consume no milk or eggs as well as no fish and meat.

Pantothenic Acid

97. Pantothenic acid is a constituent of coenzyme A, which plays a central role in fat intermediary metabolism. Deficiency diseases due to a lack of this vitamin have been produced in many species of animals and also in man. The vitamin is widely distributed in all foods. Diets in the UK usually provide 10 to 20 mg which is more than adequate.

Biotin

98. Biotin is found in living matter mostly bound to protein, probably as the active group of several carboxylases. It is widely distributed in foods and there is evidence for its synthesis in the intestine in many species, including man. Natural deficiency in adults is unknown. It is doubtful whether biotin needs to be included in the diet.

Ascorbic Acid (Vitamin C)

99. Ascorbic acid is concerned with the integrity of connective tissue constituents, particularly collagen and intercellular cement substance, but its exact mode of action is still not clear. Deficiency of the vitamin causes scurvy.

Requirements

100. The MRC Sheffield study showed that a daily intake of about 10 mg ascorbic acid could prevent or cure overt signs of scurvy in adults (Bartley, Krebs & O'Brien, 1953). This finding is supported by studies on the utilization of radioactive ascorbic acid by healthy men (Baker, personal communication).

Recommended intakes

101. There have long been two views on the need for ascorbic acid. One view maintains that an amount of the vitamin sufficient to prevent signs of deficiency,

and with a safety margin to allow for individual variation and for stresses of everyday life, can be recommended as a dietary intake. The other view is based on the concept of tissue saturation. The argument is that animal species which are able to synthesize their ascorbic acid (i.e. all except primates, the guinea pig and the fruit bat) maintain a high level of tissue saturation. For man, this requires an intake of at least 60 mg/day. There is, so far, no evidence that man derives any benefit from such a high intake of ascorbic acid.

102. USA authorities have for long advocated the desirability of tissues being kept close to saturation, and have recommended accordingly (NRC, 1964). In the UK few of us are saturated with the vitamin, but we do not appear to suffer any ill effects as a result. We therefore support the first view expressed in paragraph 101: that recommended intakes should be based on an amount sufficient to prevent signs of deficiency.

103. *Adults.* Although little is known about individual variation in requirements this may be large (Williams & Deason, 1967). Animal experiments suggest that a three-to-fourfold increase in ascorbic acid requirements occurs during periods of stress. Satisfactory wound healing may also increase the requirement. The MRC report (paragraph 100) recommended a daily intake of 30 mg as giving a reasonable safety margin for adults and we accept their figure. The available data provide no reason to alter this for the different sexes, for differences in physical activity, or for increasing age.

104. *Infants and children.* The recommended intakes for children are shown in Table 1. Human milk provides 20 to 50 mg ascorbic acid daily (WHO, 1965) and amongst breast fed infants scurvy is unknown. Artificially fed infants do not develop scurvy at levels above 7 mg/day (Van Eekelen, 1953); the recommended intake of 15 mg/day should cover their requirements with a reasonable safety margin. Newborn infants, particularly the premature, sometimes show a transient hypertyrosinaemia which might be related to ascorbic acid status (Avery, Clow, Menkes, Ramos, Scriver, Stern & Wasserman, 1967); a therapeutic daily dose of 35 mg has been recommended (Amer. Acad. Ped., 1967).

105. *Pregnancy and lactation.* Tissue levels fall during the later stages of pregnancy and therefore it is recommended that the intake should be increased to 60 mg daily. A similar recommendation is made for the period of lactation.

106. *The elderly.* There is no evidence that elderly people have a greater requirement for ascorbic acid than younger adults or that they are less able to absorb the vitamin from the diet than younger individuals. No additional intake is therefore recommended.

Sources and stability

107. Ascorbic acid is widely distributed in high but variable concentrations in fruits and vegetables. An important source in this country is potatoes. Ascorbic acid is soluble in water and large losses occur during storage, food preparation and cooking; for example, 75 per cent or more may be lost in the preparation and cooking of green vegetables. For these reasons, tables giving its content in food should be used with caution.

23

108. Retinol (vitamin A) is concerned with the integrity of mucosal surfaces, and is required in the form of its aldehyde (retinal) for vision, particularly in dim light. Night blindness, however, can arise for reasons other than lack of vitamin A in the diet, and in the UK it is rarely due to dietary deficiency. The exact mode of action of retinol other than its role in vision is still obscure. Evidence suggests that it acts in the maintenance of subcellular membranes.

Sources

109. Retinol or vitamin A is found in animal tissue; it is sometimes designated vitamin A_1 to distinguish it from the much less common vitamin A_2, dehydro-retinol, which is found mainly in the livers of freshwater fish and has about half the activity of retinol.

110. An alternative dietary source of vitamin A is provided by the intensely yellow carotenoid pigments found in plants. The most common "provitamin A" is β-carotene, the pigment which is mainly responsible for colouring the carrot. Only part of the pigment is converted into retinol due to inefficient absorption and other causes. β-carotene is present in yellow fruits, such as the apricot, and also in green vegetables. There are several other "provitamins", including α-carotene. These are converted less efficiently than β-carotene to retinol and may be taken as having half the activity of β-carotene. Carotenes contributed just under half of the total retinol equivalents provided by British diets during the years of the Second World War, but the proportion has now fallen to one-third (Greaves & Tan, 1966b).

Availability and stability

111. Retinol is easily absorbed by healthy human subjects from all its sources. The biologically active carotenoids, unlike retinol, are only sparingly soluble in fats, and in some vegetable sources may not be accompanied by enough fat to allow their efficient absorption.

112. Both retinol and carotenoids can be destroyed by exposure to oxygen, particularly at high temperatures. Under normal conditions of food storage and cooking, however, the loss of either retinol or carotene is small and can be neglected.

Units of vitamin A and carotene, and methods for expressing requirements

113. Since several substances in the diet possess vitamin A activity, we recommend that intakes be expressed in terms of "retinol equivalents". By definition, 1 μg retinol equivalent is equal to 1 μg of retinol, or 6 μg of β-carotene, or 12 μg of other biologically active carotenoids. In terms of international units, 1 μg retinol equivalent is equal to 3·33 i.u. of retinol or 10 i.u. of β-carotene. The history of vitamin A units and examples of the use of these relationships are given in Appendix 3.

Recommended intakes

114. From the findings of a long experiment on volunteers, undertaken at Sheffield during the Second World War (Hume & Krebs, 1949), the daily

vitamin A need of the human adult was assessed as 2500 i.u. of the preformed vitamin (750 μg of retinol), taking account of individual variability and allowing a margin of safety. There is no evidence that this is influenced by physical activity. The assessment of the requirement in terms of β-carotene is difficult on account of the varying absorption from food. The recommendations of Hume & Krebs (1949) to cover the derivation of carotene from different foods in a mixed diet was accepted by FAO/WHO (1967), namely that a divisor of 6 should be used in converting μg of β-carotene into μg of retinol (or a divisor of 3 for converting i.u. of carotene into i.u. of retinol). This implies that the recommended intake of β-carotene, in the complete absence of retinol from the diet, must be 4500 μg. If the vitamin A needs were to be satisfied by biologically active carotenoids other than β-carotene, the intake would have to be 9000 μg.

115. For adults we endorse the recommendations of the BMA (1950) and of FAO/WHO (1967) and recommend a daily intake of 750 μg retinol equivalents. The recommendations for children and adolescents, based on those of FAO/WHO (1967), are given in Table 1.

116. In the UK, as in many other parts of the world, body reserves of the vitamin appear to be sufficient to meet normal requirements for many months, or even years. A great excess of retinol, of the order of a hundred times the usual daily intake, is toxic both to man and experimental animals. The hypervitaminosis A so produced causes damage to bones. Great excess of carotene can cause yellow coloration of the skin, but the condition is usually harmless.

117. *Pregnancy and lactation.* The concentration of retinol in the blood decreases during pregnancy, but we do not recommend intakes sufficiently large to restore the blood retinol to the pre-pregnancy level. In lactation up to 450 μg retinol daily may be secreted in the milk and extra provision for this should be made in the mother's diet (Table 1).

Practical application of recommended intakes

118. FAO/WHO (1967) proposed that vitamin A values should be entered in tables of food composition in micrograms (μg) rather than in i.u., and under the headings of (1) retinol, (2) β-carotene, (3) other biologically active carotenoids. The contributions by carotenoids other than β-carotene, however, are usually so small in comparison to those of retinol and β-carotene, which vary greatly in their concentration in foods, that they may be neglected.

119. The following procedure is suggested for calculating the vitamin A activity of mixed diets.

 (i) Foods of animal origin, except milk and milk products, can be regarded as sources of retinol only, as carotenoids contribute rarely more than 1 per cent to the total retinol equivalents.

 (ii) In milk and milk products the carotenoids cannot be ignored as they may contribute 20 per cent or more of the total retinol equivalents. The β-carotene in milk appears to be more efficiently absorbed than that from other sources, and when milk is the major component of the diet the relationship of 2 μg β-carotene = 1 μg retinol equivalent should be used.

25

(iii) Foods derived from plants contribute only carotenoids. In green vegetables and carrots, β-carotene is the main provitamin, but the other biologically active carotenoids may be present in significant amounts. In practice, however, any overestimation resulting from including carotenoids other than β-carotene is small compared to the variations in the amounts of total carotenoids present. It therefore suffices to divide the total carotenoids by 6 to convert to retinol equivalents. However, when β-carotene is not the main carotenoid, e.g. in yellow maize where it is cryptoxanthin, a divisor of 12 is preferable. In the UK there is little maize in the diet and this consideration is not important.

Vitamin D

120. Vitamin D is represented by a group of substances of which only two are important in human nutrition. The naturally occurring vitamin is cholecalciferol (vitamin D_3), while ergocalciferol (vitamin D_2) is formed by irradiation of the plant sterol, ergosterol. Information about the exact mode of action of vitamin D is still fragmentary. It is involved in the transfer and absorption of calcium, and possibly other divalent ions, in the intestine, bones and other tissues. Deficiency of vitamin D causes rickets in the young and osteomalacia in those in whom growth has ceased.

Sources

121. Two sources of vitamin D are available: it can be obtained by exposure of the skin to sunlight, since ultra-violet rays transform 7-dehydrocholesterol present in the skin to cholecalciferol, or by ingestion from the diet.

122. Sufficient vitamin D can be derived from exposure to sunlight, but this varies with latitude and environmental conditions, and the amount available to a population cannot be assessed. Vitamin D is not found in many unfortified foods apart from fatty fish, eggs and, to a certain extent, butter, and the amount obtainable from the diet is limited unless fortified foods (e.g. margarine, infant cereals and dried milk preparations) or cod liver oil or other supplement are taken.

Units

123. We recommend that intakes be expressed in micrograms (μg), since the international unit (i.u.) of vitamin D has been defined as 0·025 μg crystalline cholecalciferol.

Recommended intakes

124. *Infants and children.* The BMA (1950) recommended 800 i.u. for children up to 2 years, while many other countries recommend 400 i.u. from infancy until growth has ceased at 18–22 years. If the vitamin D intake of infants is too high there is a danger of hypercalcaemia, since the margin between the preventive and possibly harmful doses is small. The reduction in the fortification of Welfare Foods (cod liver oil and National Dried Milk) and proprietary infant cereals, made in 1957 on the recommendation of the Joint Sub-Committee on Welfare Foods (Central and Scottish Health Services Councils, 1957) was followed by the almost complete disappearance of hypercalcaemia; the reduction itself is not thought to have affected the reported incidence of rickets. The Sub-Committee

recommended that children aged 1 to 5 years should be given 400 i.u./day. Although many children of this age may obtain substantially less dietary vitamin D than this without apparent ill health (Ministry of Health, 1968) we are reluctant to differ from the Sub-Committee's recommendations. Accordingly we recommend for children up to 5 years of age a daily intake of 10 μg cholecalciferol (400 i.u.). For older children and adolescents, in whom the contribution from sunlight is likely to be greater, we recommend an intake of 2·5 μg (100 i.u.), which may be provided without difficulty by usual diets.

125. *Adults and the elderly.* Of the requirements of adults, including the elderly, practically nothing is known. The NRC (1968), the Canadian Council on Nutrition (1964), the Swedish National Institute of Public Health (Blix, Wretlind, Bergstrom & Westin, 1967) and the BMA (1950) give no figures for men and women over the age of 22. However, the Norwegian State Nutrition Council (1958) and the Japanese Resources Council (1954) recommend 400 i.u. for adults. In the USSR tables (Yarusova, 1961) no figures for adults are listed, unless exposure to sunshine is inadequate, when 500 i.u. are recommended. Experience in the UK with elderly people confirms that if there is inadequate exposure to sunlight, there is a dietary requirement of vitamin D. As a safety measure we therefore recommend a daily intake of 2·5 μg cholecalciferol for groups of adults despite the fact that most individuals obtain all the vitamin D they need from sunlight. But for those, such as the elderly, who may be housebound and not exposed to sunlight, even more dietary vitamin D may be required. However, amounts of 2·5 μg per day appear to have a therapeutic effect in elderly patients with osteomalacia (Gough, Lloyd & Wills, 1964).

126. *Pregnancy and lactation.* The Canadian Council on Nutrition (1964) and the NRC (1964) recommend 400 i.u. for late pregnancy and lactation. In Sweden, Blix, Wretlind, Bergstrom & Westin (1967) recommend 400 i.u. for the entire period of pregnancy and lactation. The BMA (1950) recommend 400 i.u. during the first half of pregnancy, increasing thereafter to 600 i.u., and to 800 i.u. during lactation. However, we know of no evidence to support these higher figures. We therefore recommend 10 μg cholecalciferol daily throughout pregnancy and in lactation.

Vitamin E

127. Animals deficient in vitamin E develop a variety of pathological conditions, but in man no clinical syndrome has been established as a result of deficiency. Although the vitamin has been used in the treatment of a number of human conditions, including muscular dystrophy, habitual abortion, sterility, stillbirths, and skin disorders, the evidence of its effectiveness has not been convincing.

128. Vitamin E activity is found in several tocopherols. *In vitro* these substances have an antioxidant action, particularly affecting the rate of oxidation of fat, and can influence the enzymatic activity of the cell. However, it is doubtful whether these effects can explain the physiological actions of the vitamin. When intestinal absorption is impaired, low serum and tissue tocopherol levels may be found, together with increased susceptibility of erythrocytes to hydrogen peroxide. A low serum tocopherol may also be associated with increased blood and urine creatine levels, but these biochemical changes have not been related to any clinical or pathological disturbances.

27

129. Dietary vitamin E is almost certainly needed by human beings, but there is no evidence upon which a valid estimate of requirement can be based. The vitamin occurs widely in nature and is present in small quantities in many plants, the embryos of seeds, in milk and egg yolks. Most diets provide 10 mg/day or more.

Vitamin K

130. Vitamin K is essential for the clotting of the blood. It is necessary for the production of prothrombin in the liver, and may also be concerned with the synthesis of other blood clotting factors.

131. Two forms of the vitamin are found in nature, with different side-chains in their molecules, and several compounds with vitamin K activity have been synthesized; all are related to 2-methyl 1,4 naphthoquinone (menaphthone or menadione), which is a synthetic analogue soluble in fats but only slightly in water, and about twice as active as the natural forms of the vitamin. Vitamin K_1 is present in dark green vegetables such as spinach, kale and the outer leaves of cabbage, and also in cauliflower, green tomatoes, peas and cereals, but there is little in animal foods such as milk, eggs and meat. Vitamin K_2 is synthesized by bacteria, including those in the human colon; it has about three-quarters of the activity of vitamin K_1.

132. The role of the intestine in synthesizing the vitamin is not fully established, but since a primary dietary deficiency is very rare in adults, it is probable that absorption from the colon is significant. This is supported by the observations that when bacterial growth is suppressed by antibiotic therapy, there is an increased sensitivity to vitamin K antagonists (Deutsch, 1966), and that menaphthone is equally effective whether given to infants rectally or intramuscularly (Aballi, Howard & Triplett, 1966). In the newborn infant, vitamin K deficiency has been reported; before the intestinal flora become established, prothrombin and other clotting factors are present in low levels, which drop even further in the first few days of life, but rise after about the first week and gradually attain the adult values.

133. Many preparations of vitamin K, some dispersable in water, are available for therapeutic purposes to be administered either orally or parenterally, but under normal conditions a dietary deficiency of vitamin K is rarely if ever seen, and because of the variable contribution from the intestinal flora a recommended intake for the vitamin cannot be established.

Essential Fatty Acids (EFA)

134. Many species of animals develop a deficiency disease on diets lacking certain polyunsaturated fatty acids (linoleic acid, linolenic acid, arachidonic acid). A dietary supply of these acids is almost certainly required by man. However, there is no unequivocal evidence that man ever develops any deficiency disease as a result of a dietary lack; if such a condition does occur, it must be very rare. On present evidence, 1 to 2 per cent of the energy value of a diet provided by EFA meets the requirements. Diets in the UK supply many times this amount.

MINERALS

135. Of the dozen or so mineral elements known to be essential for man only three, calcium, iron and iodine, need attention. The others are widely distributed in all diets and are treated briefly at the end of this section.

Calcium

136. The adult body contains about 1200 g of calcium, 99 per cent of which is in the skeleton. The hard structure of the bones and teeth consists chiefly of phosphates of calcium. Among common foods milk and cheese are the richest sources of calcium, and together provide about 60 per cent of calcium in most diets in the UK, fortified cereal foods supplying about 20 per cent.

Adults

137. The BMA (1950) recommended 800 mg a day for adults after consideration of balance studies made chiefly in western countries where the intake of calcium is high. However, it is now well known that adaptation to a lower calcium intake occurs after a period of time, and the negative calcium balance shown at first on reducing the calcium intake below 800 mg does not necessarily mean that the body requires this amount of calcium. FAO/WHO (1962) suggested a "practical allowance" for adults of 400 to 500 mg calcium/day; this range was chosen as there appeared to be no evidence of calcium deficiency in countries where calcium intakes were of this order.

138. FAO/WHO (1962) considered that the evidence supporting the view that osteoporosis may be due to an inadequate dietary supply of calcium was not convincing. Nordin (1966), after surveying the international prevalence of osteoporosis, concluded that it occurred in old people "regardless of diet" but did not appear in young people "whatever their calcium intake". Osteoporosis develops more quickly in women than in men, and the condition becomes increasingly common with age in both sexes. Garn, Rohmann & Wagner (1967) showed no relationship between bone loss and calcium intake, and concluded that, beginning by the fifth decade in both sexes, bone loss is a general phenomenon, and progresses more than twice as fast in the female as in the male. They stated that "intakes of calcium above 1500 mg a day do not seem to be 'protective', and levels of calcium intake even below 300 mg are not demonstrably associated with bone loss". Smith (1967) found that some women lost bone despite diets rich in calcium, whereas others of similar heights and weights apparently lost no more bone through years of very low consumption of calcium; he concluded that some factor or factors other than diet were the cause of "this seemingly 'normal' or inherent bone loss". Newton-John & Morgan (1968) suggest that the amount of bone present in old age is related to the amount present in early adult life and not to subsequent calcium intake.

139. In view of the evidence that it is impossible to prevent osteoporosis with dietary calcium in adult life, there is no reason, if vitamin D is adequate, for departing from the FAO/WHO recommendation for calcium intake for adults: Table 1 sets out the upper figure in their range.

Children

140. Families with three or more children fail on average to reach the BMA (1950) recommended level of calcium intake. This has been the position for many

years, although the average intake has not fallen to less than 80 per cent of the recommended level, the lower limit of the range which has been taken as a signal for "watchful concern" (Ministry of Agriculture, Fisheries and Food, 1967). Although National Food Survey findings have been interpreted by some people to mean that these families are calcium deficient, no clinical evidence of primary calcium deficiency has been reported in the UK, or indeed anywhere in the world.

141. It is known that children in large families in the UK are smaller than their counterparts in small families, but this might be due to a number of factors, not all of them nutritional. We know of no evidence that children in countries where the calcium intake is low fail to reach full height because they are calcium deficient; addition of calcium to the diet has not resulted in improved growth.

142. The amount of bone possessed in early adult life is determined by genetic factors and physical activity and possibly also by calcium intake in childhood. If nearly 1200 g of calcium is to be provided in 20 years (paragraph 136) the average amount of calcium required to be retained during this time is 160 mg/day, the amount varying with rate of growth and body size. It is impossible to infer the required dietary intake of calcium from the tissue demand, until the extent of the variability in the efficiency of alimentary absorption is established.

143. The BMA (1950) recommendations of 1 g/day of calcium for children and 1·1 to 1·4 g/day for different ages and sexes of adolescents may be in excess of requirements. Nevertheless their retention would be justified if a high calcium intake during the growing period was needed for maximum calcification of the skeleton; and if maximum calcification of the skeleton in early adult life led to relatively large amounts of bone in old age and hence reduced the likelihood of osteoporosis. However, we are reluctant to base our recommendations on such speculation. We know of no evidence that calcium intakes greater than those suggested by FAO/WHO (1962) guard against the possibility that calcium deficiency during growth may lead to a diminished amount of bone in early adult life and thus perhaps an increased risk of osteoporosis later. We have therefore used the upper figures in the FAO/WHO range in Table 1.

Pregnancy and lactation

144. The additional calcium required for the fetus is about 30 g, and 150 to 300 mg calcium is secreted daily in the milk during lactation. Part of the extra requirement may be met by increased alimentary absorption and part from bone. We know of no evidence to justify a departure from the recommendation of FAO/WHO (1962) that 1000 to 1200 mg calcium/day during the third trimester of pregnancy and throughout lactation is a suitable amount.

Iron

145. The body of a healthy adult contains some 3 to 4 g of iron, of which approximately two-thirds is present in the red blood pigment haemoglobin and concerned with the transfer of oxygen to the tissues. In assessing dietary iron requirements a relationship is often assumed between the haemoglobin level, which is commonly taken as a measure of iron status, and the total amount of iron ingested. There is no evidence for such a relationship in the UK at the present time.

146. However, in the 1930s when iron intakes in the UK were generally lower than at present, iron deficiency was common (Davidson, Fullerton & Campbell, 1935; Orr, 1936; Fullerton, 1936) and responded to iron therapy. Many women who were living on poor diets providing less than 10 mg of iron/day were severely anaemic and suffered much ill health as a result, although dietary iron deficiency may not have been the sole cause, and gynaecological conditions may have contributed. Nowadays when most women receive 12 mg/day and additional iron during pregnancy, severe anaemia is much less common. As there is good evidence of an association between menstrual loss of iron and haemoglobin level (Elwood, Rees & Thomas, 1968), variations in menstrual losses further complicate the interpretation of observations on the diet and iron status in a community.

147. Assessments of dietary requirements have also been based on estimates of iron loss from the body (paragraph 150). However, this approach requires more precise estimates of the proportionate absorption of iron from different foods and of iron losses than have so far been practicable. Moreover, the extent of loss may itself be influenced by the amount of iron absorbed.

148. The proportion of the iron present in different foodstuffs which is absorbed. varies so much that estimates of dietary intake may be misleading. Absorption depends on the level of iron in the blood, the availabilities of iron in different foods, and the effects of other foods and nutrients, e.g. ascorbic acid (Moore, 1968; Elwood, 1968). We considered whether the dietary iron might be grouped into that from animal sources, from vegetable sources and from added iron salts; the iron content of a diet might then be expressed as "iron equivalents", using weighting factors based on the relative availabilities of iron from each source. However, at present there is not enough information about the availability of iron in different foods, and in meals of different composition, to justify such a procedure.

149. The uncertainty of the physiological value of much of the iron in the diet and ignorance of many of the factors that determine iron absorption led some of us to the view that it was premature and potentially misleading to recommend a single figure for dietary iron intake for each different category of persons shown in Table 1. Such a figure could theoretically be met from various combinations of foods, which could involve wide variations in the amount of iron actually absorbed.

150. But most of us agreed that, in spite of the difficulties in recommending figures for dietary iron intake irrespective of the type of food and knowledge about absorption, guidance should be given for the planning and interpreting of diets. It is commonly accepted that men and post-menopausal women need to absorb about 0·5 to 1 mg of iron/day, and also, that about 10 per cent of dietary iron is absorbed. On this basis, the recommended intake of iron for men and post-menopausal women is given as 10 mg/day. Menstruating women need to absorb about twice as much, but, if anaemic, are likely to absorb more than 10 per cent of their dietary iron, and we are not persuaded of the need to increase the recommended intake for women above the 12 mg recommended by the BMA (1950).

151. For children, we also retain the BMA (1950) recommendations, as set out in Table 1. The BMA (1950), a Study Group on Iron Deficiency Anaemia (WHO,

31

1959) and an Expert Group on Nutrition in Pregnancy and Lactation (WHO, 1965) each recommended that 15 mg iron daily be provided during pregnancy and lactation, and we recommend likewise.

Iodine

152. Iodine forms part of the molecule of the hormones secreted by the thyroid gland. In some areas of the world, where the water contains very little iodine, and consequently the foodstuffs produced on the land are also low in iodine, endemic goitre is present. There are other places, however, where similar amounts of dietary iodine appear sufficient to prevent goitre (Kilpatrick & Wilson, 1964). Possibly this reflects differences in the form of iodine present, or it may conceal losses during cooking; fish, for example, may lose as much as half its iodine in this way (Harrison, McFarlane, Harden & Wayne, 1965).

153. The BMA (1950) recommended intakes of 100 μg iodine daily for adults and 150 μg for children, adolescents and pregnant and nursing women. Evidence suggests that existing recommended intakes are unlikely in practice to be met in this country without iodization of salt; yet not all those who have studied the epidemiology of goitre in this country agree that iodization is indicated.

154. Small simple goitres may merely reflect a process of adaptation to intakes that are low but not inadequate, while at the other extreme the possibility exists that high intakes of iodine may exacerbate thyrotoxicoses in certain individuals. Whilst it is common to supply iodine supplements during pregnancy (Vitamin A and D tablets supplied to pregnant and lactating women under the Welfare Foods Scheme contain just under 100 μg of iodine), such supplements are likely to be ineffective in diminishing the increased thyroid clearance or the size of the goitre of pregnancy because of the prolonged period of adaptation required (Crooks, Tulloch, Turnbull, Davidsson, Skulason & Snaedal, 1967). Therefore it seems more reasonable to make recommendations applying to females in the reproductive age group than to differentiate between pregnant and non-pregnant women.

155. It is unlikely that young children or adolescents would benefit from an intake of more than 300 μg daily, and a recommendation of 150 μg daily would probably be reasonable. Similar intakes consumed by women throughout the child-bearing span would protect them during the actual period of pregnancy. Nevertheless, much more information is needed before recommended intakes can be proffered with any degree of confidence.

Sodium, Potassium and Chloride

156. The dietary intakes of these three minerals are generally more than the requirements, and the excess is readily excreted by the kidneys, provided the water intake is adequate. The daily intake of sodium is about 3 to 6 g, of potassium 2 to 4 g, and of chloride 5 to 9 g. The intakes of sodium and chloride are chiefly dependent upon the amount of salt added to food during preparation and at the table. Because some old people eat little food their diets may contain less than 2 g potassium; this may lead to potassium deficiency, especially if losses are increased by the habitual use of purgatives and diuretics.

Magnesium and Phosphorus

157. Magnesium occurs widely in foods, particularly those of plant origin, as it is a constituent of chlorophyll; a dietary deficiency of magnesium is unlikely to occur in health. The daily intake ranges from 150 to 450 mg. Dietary deficiency of phosphorus is not known to occur in man because it is present in nearly all foods. The daily intake of phosphorus is of the order of 1·2 to 2·0 g.

Fluoride

158. Fluoride is widely distributed in foods, and about 0·6 to 1·8 mg is obtained daily from food and beverages. A significant source is tea, which may provide as much as 1 mg fluoride a day. If the drinking water contains 1 part per million of fluoride these intakes are increased to about 1·2 to 3·2 mg (Longwell, 1957). A concentration of 1 part per million of fluoride in drinking water has the beneficial effect of protecting children's teeth from dental caries.

Other elements

159. Other elements known to be essential in human metabolism are copper, zinc, manganese, cobalt, selenium, molybdenum and chromium. No deficiencies of these elements have been reported among the UK population, and it must be concluded that our diet contains adequate amounts. Intakes of copper, manganese and zinc are respectively about 2 to 2·5, 5 to 10, and 10 to 15 mg/day. Cobalt, selenium, molybdenum and chromium are needed in very much smaller amounts.

160. Strontium is present in bones and teeth but has no known physiological function. It is widely distributed in foods and in drinking water.

APPENDIX 1

Body Size and Composition

by R. Passmore

1. The human body can be divided into three compartments: *the cell mass*, which consists of the actively metabolizing cells; *the extracellular supporting tissues*, which consist of the extracellular water, including the blood plasma, the collagen and other proteins in connective tissues and the bone minerals; *the energy reserve*, which consists of fat, triglycerides, present in the adipose tissue cells. The first two compartments taken together are referred to as the lean body mass.

2. The weights of the FAO reference man and woman are respectively 65 kg and 55 kg, and we have shown these in Table 1. In the USA, the NRC (1968) base their calculations on a 70 kg man and a 58 kg woman. Most figures obtained in the UK for the average weight of groups of healthy young men and women fall in between these values. The size of the body and of its different compartments is determined genetically, though the size of the energy reserve may be greatly modified by the state of nutrition. Representative values for the size of the compartments in a healthy man and woman are:

	Man		Woman	
	kg	per cent	kg	per cent
Cell mass	36	55·5	26	47·5
Extracellular supporting tissues	21	32·0	15	27·5
Energy reserve	8	12·5	14	25·0
	65	100	55	100

3. The energy reserve compartment may be as large as 20 per cent in a man and 30 per cent in a woman before the individual could be considered obese. If the compartment was as small as 5 per cent of body weight in a man or 15 per cent in a woman, the individual would certainly be thin, but not necessarily unhealthy. Indeed many athletes when in training are as thin as this.

4. The metabolism of the body takes place in the cells and the requirements of protein and of some of the vitamins are more closely related to cell mass than to body weight, surface area or any other parameter. The cell mass cannot be measured directly, but it can be calculated from measurements of total body potassium or of total body water and extracellular water. These measurements are not readily made and cannot as yet be carried out as a routine. The basal or resting metabolism is more easily measured and values can be derived from tables. Resting metabolism is closely correlated with cell mass.

5. *Normal values for resting metabolism* which we have used are:

Boys and Girls	kcal/24 hr	Men	kcal/24 hr
0 up to 1 year	400	18 up to 35 years	1600
1 up to 2 years	600	35 up to 65 years	1500
2 up to 3 years	700	65 up to 75 years	1450
3 up to 5 years	800	75 and over	1350
5 up to 7 years	900		
7 up to 9 years	1000	*Women*	
		18 up to 55 years	1300
Boys		55 up to 75 years	1200
9 up to 12 years	1200	75 and over	1100
12 up to 15 years	1400		
15 up to 18 years	1700		
Girls			
9 up to 12 years	1150		
12 up to 15 years	1400		
15 up to 18 years	1400		

The values are calculated from the body weights in Table 1, assuming a normal body composition (Durnin & Passmore, 1967). Almost identical values would be obtained, assuming figures for height, deriving the surface area from a nomogram and using one or other of the older tables (e.g. Fleisch, 1951).

6. The ratio of cell mass to extracellular supporting tissue is relatively constant in health. In consequence lean body mass is an indirect measure of cell mass. This does not apply in pathological states where there is oedema or dehydration, or to newborn infants who contain a relatively large amount of water, most of which is extracellular. By the age of about 2 years adult proportions are virtually reached. The lean body mass, like the cell mass, can be derived from laboratory measurements, such as total body water or body fat, which may be estimated by underwater weighing. Methods of determining total body water are being made more simple and the techniques for measuring skinfold thicknesses and deriving from them a value for body fat appear to be becoming more reliable. Hence it is possible that values for lean body mass may become relatively easy to obtain and that they will provide a useful standard for assessing requirements of certain nutrients.

7. The study of the composition, function and size of the compartments of the body has been developing steadily for 20 years. Passmore & Draper (1964) summarize the present position and provide a bibliography of the important papers.

APPENDIX 2

Individual Variation in Minimum Requirements for Nitrogen Balance

by J. S. Garrow

1. Sherman (1920) collected the information from 109 nitrogen balance experiments which had been made in the course of 25 separate investigations. The apparent daily protein requirement for a 70 kg man in this series ranged from the extremes of 21 to 65 g. However, this range represents variations between investigations rather than between individuals, and Sherman himself comments that some experiments may have been included which gave misleadingly high results because of too short periods on the low protein diets.

2. In the following table, Sherman's data are arranged to show the variation in requirement which has been found within any one experimental group. The table includes only 101 results, because 8 of the 109 given by Sherman were measurements on one subject only, and, therefore, do not contribute to our understanding of individual variation. The last column of the table shows that the estimated protein requirements exceeded 1·2 times the estimated requirements for their group in only 3 of the 101 subjects.

3. Two more recent investigations give similar results. Hegsted, Tsongas, Abbott & Stare (1946) estimated the requirements of 25 subjects aged 19 to 50 years. On a largely vegetable diet the standard deviation in the requirement for balance was about 6 per cent of the mean. Chan & Waterlow (1966) measured nitrogen balance in 17 Jamaican children aged 1 year. Forty balance measurements were made at various levels of intake of a milk diet, and the individual variation in the amount retained was less than 10 per cent of the average intake.

Conclusion

4. The available evidence suggests that, if the mean protein requirement for a group of people is known, an allowance of 1·2 times that mean value will cover the needs of 97 per cent of this group.

Nitrogen balance data reviewed by Sherman (1920) arranged to show variations found within the groups investigated

Author		Number of subjects in group	Protein requirements for balance per day per 70 kg subject		Number of subjects in group *not* covered by $1 \cdot 2 \times$ mean
			Mean for group	Range	
Hirschfield	(1887)	2	38·5	38–39	0
Klemperer	(1889)	2	31·5	30–33	0
Voit	(1889)	2	63	61–65	0
Siven	(1900)	2	40	37–43	0
Jaffe	(1902)	7	50	42–57	0
Chittenden	(1905)	12	52·4	40–62	0
Hindhede	(1912)	4	41·5	39–43	0
Hindhede	(1913)	8	40	31–48	0
Hindhede	(1914)	9	40·8	21–52	2
Abderhalden	(1915)	6	40·8	32–58	1
Rose	(1917)	3	40·8	37–44	0
Sherman	(1918)	8	56·7	51–60	0
Sherman	(1918)	5	53·2	52–54	0
Sherman	(1918)	16	40·4	36–46	0
Sherman	(1919)	9	39·0	33–43	0
Sherman (unpubl.)		2	47·5	44–51	0
Sherman (unpubl.)		4	33·2	32–35	0
Total		101			3

APPENDIX 3

History of Vitamin A Units and Calculation of the Vitamin A Value of Diets

by T. Moore and J. P. Greaves

1. Nearly 40 years ago crystalline β-carotene was recognized as the precursor of vitamin A in the animal body and chosen as the international standard of vitamin A activity. The size of the international unit was chosen as 0·6 μg of β-carotene.

2. When eventually pure retinol became available, and β-carotene and retinol could be compared on a weight basis, a consensus of opinion accepted 0·3 μg of the vitamin (retinol) as the biological equivalent of 0·6 μg of the provitamin (β-carotene). This relationship applied only when both retinol and β-carotene were administered to animals in low doses and in readily available form, namely in oily solution. Since retinol has half the number of carbon atoms of β-carotene and consequently about half its molecular weight, the biological equality between 0·3 μg of retinol and 0·6 μg of β-carotene might suggest that half of each carotene molecule is wasted during conversion. However, recent studies (Huang & Goodman, 1965; Goodman, Blomstrand, Werner, Huang & Shiratori, 1966; Blomstrand & Werner, 1967) indicate that both halves of the β-carotene molecule can be converted to retinol. It is therefore probable that the lower biological activity derived from β-carotene, even under the best conditions, is due to other causes, such as low absorption, transport or other factors which might influence its efficiency of utilization.

3. In view of the greater stability of retinylacetate and because it is more easily obtainable in pure, crystalline form than the free alcohol, the acetate ester of retinol was chosen as reference substance for the international unit. To allow for the increased molecular weight, the unit was defined as 0·344 μg of retinylacetate.

Calculations

4. The Panel has recommended (paragraph 113) that vitamin A intakes should be expressed in terms of retinol equivalents, and have defined 1 μg retinol equivalent as being equal to:

        1 μg retinol

or 6 μg β-carotene

or 12 μg other biologically active carotenoids

or   3·33 i.u. retinol $(=\frac{1}{0.3})$

or 10 i.u. β-carotene $(=3·33 \times 3)$.

5. These relationships are based on the definition of the international unit of retinol (1 i.u. retinol = 0·3 μg retinol = 0·344 μg retinylacetate) and the factor of 3 chosen for converting i.u. of β-carotene into i.u. of retinol. Other factors have sometimes been chosen: for example, the NRC (1964) adopted a factor of 2. Care must therefore be exercised in interpreting reported intakes to ensure that the adopted practices are understood (Greaves & Tan, 1966b). It is similarly essential to know whether the values given for vegetables in food tables are gross provitamin values, or whether they have been already divided by a factor to allow for the inefficient utilization of provitamins.

38

6. In reporting actual dietary intakes it is still desirable to give both the retinol and β-carotene intakes rather than just the intake of retinol equivalents, since the suggested correction for the efficiency of utilization of β-carotene is still tentative.

7. There are several possibilities for calculations which depend on the information available:

(i) Amounts of retinol and β-carotene may be given in μg.

The number of retinol equivalents in a diet containing 500 μg retinol and 1500 μg β-carotene $= 500 + \dfrac{1500}{6} = 750$ μg.

(ii) Amounts may be given in i.u.

The number of retinol equivalents in a diet containing 1666 i.u. retinol and 2500 i.u. β-carotene $= \dfrac{1666}{3 \cdot 33} + \dfrac{2500}{10} = 500 + 250 = 750$ μg.

(iii) Retinol may be given in i.u. and β-carotene in μg.

This situation would arise for example from use of the food composition tables of McCance & Widdowson (1967). The number of retinol equivalents in a diet containing 1666 i.u. retinol and 1500 μg β-carotene $= \dfrac{1666}{3 \cdot 33} + \dfrac{1500}{6} = 750$ μg.

REFERENCES

Aballi, A. J., Howard, C. E. & Triplett, R. F., 1966. Absorption of vitamin K from the colon in the newborn infant. *J. Pediat.*, **68**, 305–308.

American Academy of Pediatrics, Committee on Nutrition, 1967. Proposed changes in food and drug administration regulations concerning formula products and vitamin-mineral dietary supplements for infants. *Pediatrics*, **40**, 916–922.

Ashworth, A. & Harrower, A. D. B., 1967. Protein requirements in tropical countries: nitrogen losses in sweat and their relation to nitrogen balance. *Br. J. Nutr.*, **21**, 833–843.

Avery, M. E., Clow, C. L., Menkes, J. H., Ramos, A., Scriver, C. R., Stern, L. & Wasserman, B. P., 1967. Transient tyrosinemia of the newborn: dietary and clinical aspects. *Pediatrics*, **39**, 378–384.

Bartley, W., Krebs. H. A. & O'Brien, J. R. P., 1953. Vitamin C requirement of human adults. *Spec. Rep. Ser. med. Res. Coun., Lond.*, **280**. London, HMSO.

Blix, G., Wretlind, A., Bergstrom, S. & Westin, S. I., 1967. *The national diet in Sweden and a programme for its revision.* Stockholm, National Institute of Public Health.

Blomstrand, R. & Werner, B., 1967. Studies of intestinal absorption of radioactive carotene and vitamin A in man. *Scand. J. clin. Lab. Invest.*, **19**, 339–345.

Bransby, E. R. & Fothergill, J. E., 1954. Diets of young children. *Br. J. Nutr.*, **8**, 195–204.

Bricker, M. L., Shively, R. F., Smith, J. M., Mitchell, H. H. & Hamilton, T. S., 1949. The protein requirements of college women on high cereal diets with observations on the adequacy of short balance periods. *J. Nutr.*, **37**, 163–183.

British Medical Association, 1950. *Report of the Committee on Nutrition.* London, British Medical Association.

Bro-Rasmussen, F., 1958. The riboflavin requirement of animals and man and associated metabolic relations. Part II: Relation of requirement to the metabolism of protein and energy. *Nutr. Abstr. Rev.*, **28**, 369–386.

Butterworth, C. E., 1968. The availability of food folate. *Br. J. Haemat.*, **14**, 339–343.

Canadian Council on Nutrition, 1964. Dietary standard for Canada. *Can. Bull. Nutr.*, **6**, 1–76.

Central and Scottish Health Services Councils, Standing Medical Advisory Committees 1957,. *Report of the Joint Sub-Committee on Welfare Foods.* London, HMSO.

Chan, H. & Waterlow, J. C., 1966. The protein requirement of infants at the age of about one year. *Br. J. Nutr.*, **20**, 775–782.

Chaudhuri, D. K. & Kodicek, E., 1949. Fluorimetric estimation of nicotinamide in biological materials. *Biochem. J.*, **44**, 343–348.

Chittenden, R. H., 1905. *Physiological economy in nutrition, with special reference to the minimal proteid requirement of the healthy man: an experimental study.* London, Heinemann.

Clegg, K. M., 1963. Bound nicotinic acid in dietary wheaten products. *Br. J. Nutr.*, **17**, 325–329.

Crooks, J., Tulloch, M. I., Turnbull, A. C., Davidsson, D., Skulason, T. & Snaedal, G., 1967. Comparative incidence of goitre in pregnancy in Iceland and Scotland. *Lancet*, ii, 625–627.

Darke, S. J., 1960. The cutaneous loss of nitrogen compounds in African adults. *Br. J. Nutr.*, **14**, 115–119.

Davidson, L. S. P., Fullerton, H. W. & Campbell, R. M., 1935. Nutritional iron-deficiency anaemia. *Br. med. J.*, ii, 195–198.

Deutsch, E., 1966. Vitamin K in medical practice: adults. *Vitams Horm.*, **24**, 665–678.

Durnin, J. V. G. A., 1966. Age, physical activity and energy expenditure. *Proc. Nutr. Soc.*, **25**, 107–113.

Durnin, J. V. G. A. & Lonergan, M., 1968. Energy requirements in fourteen year old adolescents. *J. Physiol., London.*, **196**, 46P–47P.

Durnin, J. V. G. A. & Passmore, R., 1967. *Energy, work and leisure.* London, Heinemann.

Elwood, P. C., 1968. Some epidemiological problems of iron deficiency anaemia. *Proc. Nutr. Soc.*, **27**, 14–23.

Elwood, P. C., Rees, G. and Thomas, J. D. R., 1968. Community study of menstrual iron loss and its association with iron deficiency anaemia. *Br. J. prev. soc. Med.*, **22**, 127-131.

Fleisch, A., 1951. Le métabolisme basal standard et sa détermination au moyen du "metabo-calculator". *Helv. med. Acta*, **18**, 23–44.

Fomon, S. J., 1960. Comparative study of adequacy of protein from human milk and cow's milk in promoting nitrogen retention by normal full-term infants. *Pediatrics, Springfield*, **26**, 51–61.

Fomon, S. J., 1967. *Infant nutrition*. Philadelphia and London, W. B. Saunders.

Food and Agriculture Organization, 1957. Calorie requirements: report of the Second Committee on Calorie Requirements. *FAO nutr. Stud.*, **15**.

Food and Agriculture Organization and World Health Organization, 1962. Calcium requirements: report of an FAO/WHO Expert Group. *FAO Nutr. Mtg Rep. Ser.*, **30** and *Tech. Rep. Ser. Wld Hlth Organ.*, **230**.

Food and Agriculture Organization and World Health Organization, 1965. Protein requirements: report of a Joint FAO/WHO Expert Group. *FAO Nutr. Mtg Rep. Ser.*, **37** and *Tech. Rep. Wld Hlth Organ.*, **301**.

Food and Agriculture Organization and World Health Organization, 1967. Requirements of Vitamin A, thiamine, riboflavine and niacin: report of a joint FAO and WHO Expert Group. *FAO Nutr. Mtg Rep. Ser.*, **41** and *Tech. Rep. Ser. Wld Hlth Org.*, **362**.

Fowke, H. M., 1945. Discussion. In: The organization of large-scale surveys, by M. Greenwood. *Proc. Nutr. Soc.*, **3**, 28–30.

Fullerton, H. W., 1936. Hypochromic anaemias of pregnancy and the puerperium. *Br. med. J.*, ii, 577–581.

Garn, S. M., Rohmann, G. C. & Wagner, B., 1967. Bone loss as a general phenomenon in man. *Fedn Proc. Fedn Am. Socs exp. Biol.*, **26**, 1729–1736.

Goodman, D. S., Blomstrand, R., Werner, B., Huang, H. S. & Shiratori, T., 1966. The intestinal absorption and metabolism of vitamin A and β-carotene in man. *J. clin. Invest.*, **45**, 1615–1623.

Gough, K. R., Lloyd, O. C. & Wills, M. R., 1964. Nutritional osteomalacia. *Lancet*, ii, 1261–1264.

Greaves, J. P. & Hollingsworth, D. F., 1964. Protein supplies in the United Kingdom. In: Requirements of man for protein, Appendix 5. *Rep. publ. Hlth med. Subj., London.*, **111**, 63–72. London, HMSO.

Greaves, J. P. & Tan, J., 1966a. The amino acid pattern of the British diet. *Nutrition, Lond.*, **20**, 112–115.

Greaves, J. P. & Tan, J., 1966b. Vitamin A and carotene in British and American diets. *Br. J. Nutr.*, **20**, 819–824.

Harper, L. J., 1960. Description of metabolic studies. *Fedn Proc. Fedn Am. Socs. exp. Biol.*, **19**, 1007–1008.

Harries, J. M., Hobson, E. A. & Hollingsworth, D. F., 1962. Individual variations in energy expenditure and intake. *Proc. Nutr. Soc.*, **21**, 157–178.

Harrison, M. T., McFarlane, S., Harden, R. McG. & Wayne, E., 1965. Nature and availability of iodine in fish. *Am. J. clin. Nutr.*, **17**, 73–77.

Hegsted, D. M., Tsongas, A. G., Abbott, D. B. & Stare, F. J., 1946. Protein requirements of adults. *J. Lab. clin. Med.*, **31**, 261–284.

Huang, H. S. & Goodman, D. S., 1965. Vitamin A and carotenoids. I. Intestinal absorption and metabolism of 14C labelled vitamin A alcohol and β-carotene in the rat. *J. biol. Chem.*, **240**, 2839–2844.

Hume, E. M. & Krebs, H. A., 1949. Vitamin A requirements of human adults. *Spec. Rep. Ser. med. Res. Coun., Lond.*, **264**. London, HMSO.

Hytten, F. E. & Leitch, I., 1964. *The physiology of human pregnancy*. Oxford, Blackwell.

Hytten, F. E. & Thomson, A. M., 1961. Nutrition in the lactating woman. In: *Milk: the mammary gland and its secretion*, edited by S. K. Kon and A. T. Cowie. New York and London, Academic Press, vol. 2, pp. 3–46.

James, W. H., 1960. Nitrogen balance. *Fedn Proc. Fedn Am. Socs. exp. Biol.*, **19**, 1009–1011.

Japanese Resources Council, 1954. Report No. 19. Cited by Young, 1964.

Kilpatrick, R. & Wilson, G. M., 1964. Simple non-toxic goitre. In: *The thyroid gland*. Vol. II, edited by R. Pitt-Rivers and W. R. Trotter. London, Butterworth, pp. 88–111.

Kodicek, E., 1962. Nicotinic acid and the pellagra problem. *Biblthca "Nutr. Dieta"*, **4**, 109–127.

Longwell, J., 1957. Chemical and technical aspects. In: Symposium on fluoridation of public water. *R. Soc. Hlth J.*, **77**, 361–374.

McCance, R. A. & Widdowson, E. M., 1967. The composition of foods. *Spec. Rep. Ser. med. Res. Coun., Lond.*, **297**. London, HMSO.

Mayer, J. & Bullen, B., 1964. Nutrition and athletics. In: *Proceedings of the Sixth International Congress of Nutrition, Edinburgh*, 1963, edited by C. F. Mills and R. Passmore. Edinburgh and London, Livingstone, pp. 27–39.

Miller, A. T., 1968. *Energy metabolism*. Oxford, Blackwell Scientific Publications.

Miller, D. S. & Payne, P. R., 1961. Problems in the prediction of protein values of diets: the use of food composition tables. *J. Nutr.*, **74**, 413–419.

Ministry of Agriculture, Fisheries and Food, 1967. *Household food consumption and expenditure: 1965. Annual Report of the National Food Survey Committee*. London, HMSO.

Ministry of Agriculture, Fisheries and Food, 1968. *Household food consumption and expenditure: 1966. Annual Report of the National Food Survey Committee*. London, HMSO.

Ministry of Health, 1964. Requirements of man for protein. *Rep. publ. Hlth med. Subj., Lond.*, **111**. London, HMSO.

Ministry of Health, 1968. A pilot survey of nutrition of young children in 1963. *Rep. publ. Hlth med. Subj., Lond.*, **118**. London, HMSO.

Moore, C. V., 1968. The absorption of iron from foods. In: *Occurrence, causes and prevention of nutritional anaemias. Symposia of the Swedish Nutrition Foundation, VI, August*, 1967, edited by G. Blix. Stockholm, Almquist and Wiksell.

National Research Council, 1964. *Recommended dietary allowances: a report of the Food and Nutrition Board*. 6th rev. ed. (National Academy of Sciences and National Research Council Publication, No. 1146) Washington, D.C., National Academy of Sciences.

National Research Council, 1968. *Recommended dietary allowances: a report of the Food and Nutrition Board*. 7th rev. ed. (National Academy of Sciences and National Research Council Publication, No. 1694) Washington, D.C., National Academy of Sciences.

Newton-John, H. F. & Morgan, D. B., 1968. Osteoporosis: disease or senescence? *Lancet*, i, 232–233.

Nordin, B. E. C., 1966. International patterns of osteoporosis. *Clin. Orthop.*, **45**, 17–30.

Norwegian State Nutrition Council, 1958. *Evaluation of nutrition requirements*. In Norwegian; cited by Young, 1964.

Orr, J. B., 1937. *Food, health and income*. London, Macmillan.

Passmore, R. & Draper, M. H., 1964. The chemical anatomy of the human body. In: *Biochemical disorders in human disease*, 2nd edition, edited by R. H. S. Thompson and E. J. King. London, Churchill.

Sherman, H. C., 1920. Protein requirements of maintenance in man and nutritive efficiency of bread protein. *J. biol. Chem.*, **41**, 97–109.

Sirbu, E. R., Margen, S. & Calloway, D. H., 1967. Effect of reduced protein intake on nitrogen loss from the human integument. *Am. J. clin. Nutr.*, **20**, 1158–1165.

Smith, R. W., 1967. Dietary and hormonal factors in bone loss. *Fedn Proc. Fedn Am. Socs exp. Biol.*, **26**, 1737–1746.

Tanner, J. M., Whitehouse, R. H. & Takaishi, M., 1966. Standards from birth to maturity for height, weight, height velocity, and weight velocity: British children, 1965. Part 2. *Archs Dis. Childh.*, **41**, 613–635.

Van Eekelen, M., 1953. The occurrence of vitamin C in foods. *Proc. Nutr. Soc.*, **12**, 228–252.

Widdowson, E. M., 1947. A study of individual children's diets. *Spec. Rep. Ser. med. Res. Coun., Lond.*, **257**. London, HMSO.

Widdowson, E. M. & Dickerson, J. W. T., 1964. Chemical composition of the body. In: *Mineral metabolism*, vol. IIa, edited by C. L. Comar and F. Bronner. New York, Academic Press, pp. 2–247.

Williams, R. J. & Deason, G., 1967. Individuality in vitamin C needs. *Proc. natn. Acad. Sci.*, **57**, 1638–1641.

World Health Organization, 1959. Iron deficiency anaemia: report of a study group. *Tech. Rep. Ser. Wld Hlth Org.*, **182**.

World Health Organization, 1965. Nutrition in pregnancy and lactation: report of a WHO Expert Committee. *Tech. Rep. Ser. Wld Hlth Org.*, **302**.

Yarusova, N. S., 1961. *Vopr. Pitaniya*, **20**, 3. Cited by Young, 1964.

Young, E. G., 1964. Dietary standards. In: *Nutrition*, vol. II, edited by G. H. Beaton and E. W. McHenry. New York, Academic Press, pp. 299–350.

Printed in England for Her Majesty's Stationery Office by Galliard (Printers) Ltd, Great Yarmouth
3369 Dd 290586 K22 1/76